The Perimenopause Solution

About the authors

Emma Bardwell is a registered nutritionist and member of the British Menopause Society. Her evidence-based approach, coupled with an ongoing interest in perimenopause and menopause, has made her one of the go-to names in women's health. Emma combines the most up-to-date research with a 360-degree approach, focusing on diet, lifestyle, stress reduction and exercise, to help women overcome their symptoms. Emma is deeply anti-fad and doesn't care for restriction, believing in positive rather than perfect nutrition. She regularly contributes to publications such as *Red* magazine, Sheerluxe and Sweaty Betty. You can connect with her on Instagram @emma.bardwell or online at www.emmabardwell.com.

Dr Shahzadi Harper is an innovative modern menopause and women's wellbeing doctor with a holistic and medical approach. She believes in the early management of the symptoms of perimenopause and menopause and understands how our hormones affect not only our physical health, but also our mental wellbeing. Dr Harper is not afraid to discuss issues that other doctors may shy away from such as libido, vaginal dryness, ageing and sex. She's on a mission to empower women of all backgrounds and ethnicities to look and feel their best.

The Perimenopause Solution

Take control of your hormones
before they take control of you

By Dr Shahzadi Harper
and Emma Bardwell

Vermilion
LONDON

Vermilion, an imprint of Ebury Publishing,
20 Vauxhall Bridge Road,
London SW1V 2SA

Vermilion is part of the Penguin Random House group of companies
whose addresses can be found at global.penguinrandomhouse.com

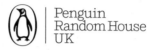

Penguin
Random House
UK

First published by Vermilion in 2021

www.penguin.co.uk

A CIP catalogue record for this book is available from the British Library

ISBN 9781785043642

Typeset in 10/15 pt Berndal LT Std
by Integra Software Services Pvt. Ltd, Pondicherry

Printed and bound in Great Britain by Clays Ltd, Elcograf S.p.A.

The authorised representative in the EEA is Penguin Random House
Ireland, Morrison Chambers, 32 Nassau Street, Dublin D02 YH68.

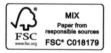

Penguin Random House is committed to a
sustainable future for our business, our readers
and our planet. This book is made from Forest
Stewardship Council® certified paper.

For our daughters.

And to all the women feeling lost,
confused and invisible.
It's time to take back control.

CONTENTS

A New Beginning

In our respective jobs – a nutritionist and a doctor, both specialising in women's health – we talk about 'perimenopause' day in, day out. In fact, it often feels like we're on repeat. Occasionally we get this niggle that people are sick of us listing symptoms and talking about the long-term risk factors of hormone deficiency. Yet after every event, every social media post, every article, every podcast, we are besieged by women clamouring to ask questions, share stories and recount experiences. And the thrust of the conversation is always the same: we had no idea this was happening to us.

Lack of understanding, including in the medical profession, is rife when it comes to perimenopause. Of late, the world is much better at talking about pregnancy, periods, postnatal depression and mental health, but there is a dearth of straight-talking, no-nonsense, evidence-based information when it comes to perimenopause. Yes, there's an unprecedented amount of noise on the subject, with people often nebulously lumping everything together under the umbrella of 'menopause', but so little of what's out there is engaging, reliable or shines a light on the most crucial part of the transition. We decided that needed to change and so *The Perimenopause Solution* was born.

How this book will help you

The Perimenopause Solution provides answers to the questions we get asked online and in clinic every day, the ones we even asked ourselves in perimenopause. Our hope is that it will liberate you from the tyranny (and expense) of unsubstantiated claims, fad diets and sham therapies. We want it to cut through the confusion and make perimenopause a much simpler and better understood process. Our hope is that, by stripping perimenopause down to its basic parts, you will get a firm grip of what's happening in your body, understand how to manage it better and turn it to your advantage. Perimenopause can be hard work – especially if you're unprepared for it – but it's not insurmountable. In fact, we'd go as far as saying it's your body's way of signalling that something needs to change. Your old ways no longer serve you; it's time to pivot.

Hormones are complicated. Our mutual interest in women's health means we get that more than most. As much as we both enjoy exploring research and bringing truths to the public, the best bit about our jobs is that we get the chance to sit down with women, listen to their worries and empower them to take control of their health. Much of what women talk to us about stems from sensationalist headlines, scaremongering on social media and mixed messages from unqualified sources. Because perimenopause is still shrouded in a fair amount of secrecy and shame, there's an unprecedented number of myths being peddled. This book turns all that on its head.

As you'll read in Chapter 1, your experience of perimenopause is based on many things, not least your socioeconomic background. If you're not getting the support you need from your doctor, private treatment is available but is outside many women's means. *The Perimenopause Solution* is as close to a private consultation as you can get without actually booking an appointment. What's more, it affords you insights from not one, but two, qualified specialists.

Science informs the way both of us practise, but we're very open to new ideas and approaches. Unlike some of its peers, our book is predicated on evidence-backed research brought to life through nearly three decades of combined clinical practice. We refer to studies and research throughout, but also weave in the experiences of real-life women and tips that we've found to be helpful, both personally and professionally. When something is anecdotal or doesn't have research to back it up yet, we tell you so. More than anything we wanted to create a book that's practical, so each chapter contains bullet point tips, nuggets of actionable advice, and ends with a summary of the most salient points – perfect if you're tired or feeling a bit foggy and haven't got the energy to read every word of every chapter.

Every woman goes through perimenopause, but her experience of that journey will be unique to her. Individualised treatment is crucial, but is outside the scope of a book so we've given you as much information as we can to enable you to tailor your approach to your own personal symptoms and experience.

How to use this book

There are three parts to *The Perimenopause Solution*:

Part 1 – Health: discover the wide range of symptoms you might experience – not just hot flushes – and understand why perimenopause can be such an individual experience.

Part 2 – Life: learn about the environment that shapes your experience of perimenopause, and how your work life and relationships might be affected.

Part 3 – Diet: become informed about how nutrition plays a key part in a healthy perimenopause and learn how to make the right food choices to maximise your health.

We suggest exploring (maybe even highlighting) the chapters and topics that feel most relevant to you, and referring back to them frequently. Your journey will morph and change along the way, so you may find that other sections become more relevant later down the line. We are both advocates of hormone therapy (HRT); it is the gold standard treatment for many perimenopause symptoms and for this reason we've dedicated an entire chapter to it and you will find references to it peppered throughout. However, HRT is only one part of the jigsaw, so we explore lifestyle, nutrition and alternative medical approaches in depth for your consideration.

You will no doubt have come across the narrative that perimenopause marks the death of youth, the end of life as you know it. It's time to knock those tired old tropes on the head once and for all. The only endings we're interested in are the end of confusion; the end of stoically wading through life; the end of feeling flattened, invisible and joyless; the end of shame. Perimenopause can be the start of a pretty wild journey but, be assured, you're nowhere near the end. In many ways, you're just beginning.

Right, we've got a lot of ground to cover, so let's dive in.

PART 1

Health

CHAPTER 1

Understanding Perimenopause

Let's change the conversation and see this time in your life through a fresh new lens.

So, what exactly is meant by perimenopause, menopause and post-menopause? In this chapter, we'll define these stages and outline what to expect at each one. We don't want you to have to 'put up' with symptoms; we want to empower you and start a different kind of conversation about this life stage. By being aware of your symptoms and being informed, we hope you can make positive choices that are right for you and optimise your perimenopause experience, seeing it in a different, more positive light.

Maria's story

I first noticed something wasn't quite right when I was around 47. I'd always been positive and confident, and I was renowned for being sharp and 'on it' at work. I gradually found it difficult to keep up with the younger women in the office and I wasn't performing well in meetings. I was having difficulty sleeping and gaining weight, which made me self-conscious in my image-obsessed office. My husband is five years younger than me and, although he hadn't said anything, I was noticing my age more than ever. I didn't feel sexy or sexual – overall, I just wasn't myself, but I couldn't put my finger on the cause. Like many women I was juggling parenthood and the pressures of work, so I put it down to that, but gradually these micro-changes chipped away at my self-esteem and confidence. I eventually saw my doctor who said, 'Your periods are still regular, so I don't think it's anything to do with the menopause. Maybe you're just a bit depressed.'

In our jobs as a doctor and a nutritionist, we often see women like Maria, who invariably tell us a slightly different version of the same story. They're overwhelmingly tired and unable to concentrate at work. Many of them are working in high-powered jobs. Their sex drives are depleted, but they don't feel they can talk to anyone about it. They say something like, 'I look and feel ten years older than I did six months ago, and it's getting me down.'

The clarity and zest that has defined their professional – and personal – lives feels as though it has disappeared, like air rapidly escaping from a punctured balloon. More often than not, they say, 'I don't know why, but I just don't feel like me. I don't know where I've gone.' Then, in the same breath, 'But I've got to keep going: with my job, my relationship, my life. The cogs have to keep turning.'

What Maria, and so many other women like her, haven't realised is that they're perimenopausal. The combination of lifestyle and health symptoms tell us as much – no blood tests required. For many women like Maria it can come as quite a shock to be told that they are 'perimenopausal'. That's for older women, isn't it? Women who are grey, moody and having hot flushes, not someone as young as me? Many women quite rightly don't see or perceive themselves like their mothers, so there can be a lot of 'menopause deniers'. It's not sexy and the narrative around a menopausal woman can be quite negative, so who would want to be part of that 'club'.

You might be perimenopausal, suspect you are, or at least be curious about what the phrase means, and how it relates to your life. 'Menopause' is being discussed in more open forums, but so many people don't *understand* peri-menopause. A combination of misinformation and, frankly, shame-induced silence, means perimenopause – arguably the most important stage of the process – is still a grey area.

Perimenopause, menopause and post-menopause explained

Most people use menopause as a byword, an umbrella term, for the time in a woman's life that encompasses perimeno-pause, menopause and post-menopause. In some ways, that's helpful, because we tend to understand and acknow-ledge the term 'menopause', whereas not everybody's heard of perimenopause. But perimenopause is the most important stage to get to grips with because that's when the majority of symptoms occur. In fact, what many women call 'menopause' is actually perimenopause. Technically, 'peri' means 'around', so perimenopause means 'around the menopause'.

Before we see them, many women with perimenopausal symptoms have already been through the wringer with their doctor. The stories they tell about their medical journey make us feel incredibly frustrated. One woman said she'd been to her doctor to discuss her symptoms seven times in seven months, and no one had joined up the dots. Others, like Maria, are asked if they have their period, and when they say they do, they're dismissed, or told they're depressed and given antidepressants.

Many doctors aren't trained in the menopause and with standard appointments lasting ten minutes, there's no time to explore the nuances of how the 34-plus officially recognised symptoms (see page 23) of the perimenopause might manifest in a woman's life. Besides, women – and many doctors – don't even consider the idea that physical and psychological symptoms in women could be hormone-related. In their medical training they may have never had one whole lecture dedicated to menopause, yet attended many on pregnancy, periods and fertility. Thankfully the landscape is now changing as more women are speaking up and speaking out.

At school, we're taught about what happens when a woman's period begins, but until 2020 there was no such class for when the menstrual cycle is coming to its end. So, here's a brief but necessary biology lesson …

Perimenopause

First, let's rewind. When we are born, we have two million eggs in our ovaries. By puberty, the number is down to about 300,000–500,000 eggs because of natural apoptosis, i.e. normal, controlled cell death. Then during every menstrual cycle an egg is released, and if it doesn't get fertilised by sperm we have a period, usually regularly and monthly.

At puberty, our ovaries kick into action and start to produce the hormones oestrogen and progesterone, which allow our breasts, hips and pubic hair to develop. These hormones govern our menstrual cycle, but once we enter our 40s, the levels of oestrogen and progesterone begin to fluctuate and naturally decline.

Throughout this time, we may still get our periods, but they might get shorter and our overall cycle might too. For example, if you normally have a 30-day cycle, it may decrease to 26 days. You might notice that you miss the odd period, they become super-heavy, or unusually light, and it can vary from month to month. These changes happen because our ovaries are no longer producing the hormones oestrogen and progesterone at the same levels that they used to; in fact, the levels are declining gradually and are at almost zero by the time most women are 55 years old. Changes to our periods can be one of the first signs of perimenopause, but that isn't true for all women and it's by no means the only indicator. Oestrogen, especially, is what makes us feel good, and having less of it can cause joint pain, hot flushes, pelvic floor and bladder issues, such as urinary leaks, low libido, vaginal atrophy (see page 112) and dryness, and more. That's some list!

If you think back to a time when you had regular periods, you might have noticed that around mid-cycle, often around day 14, you felt like the best, happiest, most energised version of yourself. That's because at that point your oestrogen levels were peaking. So, when oestrogen starts to decline and we enter perimenopause, we often don't feel on top of the world, which is why mood changes are a key symptom of perimenopause. Most of the women we see are in their 40s, but have had perimenopausal symptoms for a while.

It's key to point out, though, that each month, the levels of hormone production can fluctuate, which is why the symptoms of perimenopause fluctuate too. The consistent cycle our bodies used to follow has been disrupted, which is why, during perimenopause, some days we'll feel fine, and others, not so fine. A lot of women (and, frankly, some doctors) think because they've still got periods, they can't possibly be perimenopausal, but they could be. This time can be when symptoms are at their worst, yet remain untreated, because the presence of a period confuses people into believing that they can't be perimenopausal yet.

Menopause and post-menopause

As already mentioned, during perimenopause, you'll still have your menstrual cycle – whether it's shorter, longer or irregular – and that is the key difference between perimenopause and menopause. The very presence of a period – in whatever form – means you haven't yet reached menopause. Technically, menopause simply means your last menstrual period. It's a retrospective diagnosis that can only be given after a year of no periods. Only then can you look back on your last period, and say, 'Okay, that was my menopause.'

Post-menopause is after this point, when you've had no periods for at least a year. Although at this stage you're officially 'post-menopausal', you probably will still be symptomatic because your hormone levels are still declining.

There's no one-size-fits-all perimenopause

You often hear there are 34 symptoms of perimenopause, but we'd wager there are many more. The challenge is joining the dots of those symptoms together to discover you don't just feel tired, or flat, or overweight, in isolation. They're all connected. On page 287 you'll find the symptoms questionnaire we use, and I would invite you to look at that and fill it in.

There's no one-size-fits-all set of symptoms that define perimenopause. It's a combination. And if your blood test comes back normal, you might think you can't possibly be in perimenopause. What you need to know is this: it's not about the numbers; it's about how you feel. During

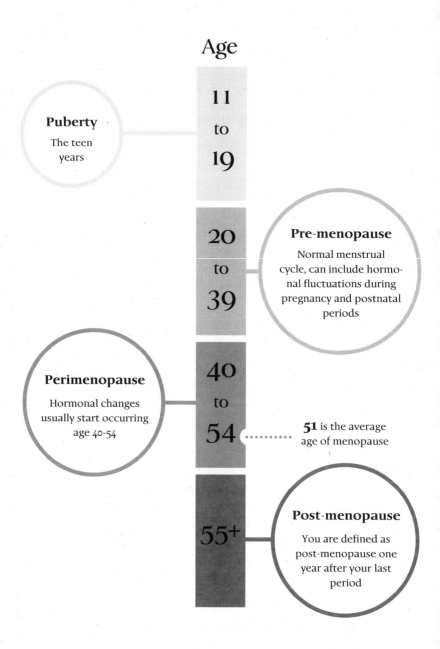

Age

Puberty

The teen years

11 to 19

20 to 39

Pre-menopause

Normal menstrual cycle, can include hormonal fluctuations during pregnancy and postnatal periods

Perimenopause

Hormonal changes usually start occurring age 40-54

40 to 54

51 is the average age of menopause

55+

Post-menopause

You are defined as post-menopause one year after your last period

WOMEN'S HORMONE TIMELINE

perimenopause, hormone levels can vary almost on a daily basis, so, in short, it's about *you* and *your* symptoms – the way you're feeling and not just the blood test levels.

In the UK, the National Institute of Health and Care Excellence (NICE) guidelines state if you're a woman aged 45 or over, you don't have to have blood tests to diagnose perimenopause; your symptoms are enough. And if you do have a blood test, then it's usually to measure your FSH (follicle stimulating hormone) level, which helps stimulate your ovaries to produce oestrogen and regulate your menstrual cycle. A high level can be an indicator of perimenopause; you can still be classified as perimenopausal if the level is normal but you have symptoms. So, don't get hung up on test results – if you're a woman over the age of 45, you've got symptoms, and you're not feeling yourself, we'd say you're in perimenopause until proven otherwise. And if you're under 45 and feeling this way, then it is probably perimenopause and now is the time to ask your doctor for some blood tests/ investigations as there are some conditions that can mimic perimenopause, such as nutritional deficiencies, thyroid disorders, chronic fatigue and fibromyalgia, which are also more frequent in midlife.

When women like Maria (see page 6) recount their stories and symptoms, we listen while they open up because perimenopause isn't talked about enough. You might think you're an anomaly, that you are the only one who is not feeling in control of your body. Feel assured that what you're going through is very normal and many women around 40 years of age are going through exactly the same thing right now. As we'll see in Part 2, perimenopausal symptoms have an impact on every aspect of your life – home, work, relationships, family, friends – so it is important to recognise and acknowledge this important life stage.

Factors that can affect perimenopause

Your ethnic background, socioeconomic status, lifestyle and medical history will all have an impact on how you experience the perimenopause. And if the dominant narrative suggests there's only one set of symptoms (those experienced by a certain type of woman) and you don't fit that demographic, you might struggle to recognise the perimenopause in yourself. Perimenopause and menopause will affect every woman, so it's key that nobody feels excluded from a dialogue which is already swamped in stigma.

We need to be aware that women of different backgrounds may present with different symptoms at different ages and stages, because it's not all mood swings and hot flushes. By growing your awareness of how *you* are likely to experience perimenopause based on *your* demographic, you'll be more likely to understand what's happening and better able to advocate for yourself when it comes to seeking medical help. It might sound strange but, believe it or not, some doctors might not be *au fait* with some of the lesser-known symptoms either.

Stressful life events, crash diets, smoking, IVF treatment, bereavement, childbirth, and having less money and education can also cause you to enter perimenopause earlier. Yes, you read that right: how affluent you are may impact your experience of perimenopause. Research shows that less well-off women are more likely to have more medical issues, be more overweight, smoke more and drink more alcohol; all factors that increase the likelihood of having hot flushes and night sweats.

Women of different ethnicities have different symptoms, too. South Asian women tend to go through perimenopause a bit earlier, with symptoms of fatigue, joint pains, vaginal atrophy (see page 112), dryness, pelvic floor issues like peeing when coughing and sneezing, and bodily aches and pains. So, if you're of South Asian origin and you keep going to your doctor with urinary tract infections or thrush, it could be because you're in perimenopause, while Black women may experience more hot flushes and night sweats.

There's also the influence of your medical history. Women who suffer with premenstrual syndrome (PMS) will have more, and usually more severe, perimenopausal symptoms.

Don't hold too much store in what age your mother went through menopause for an indicator of yours because we lead very different lives to our mothers, but if your mother went through an early menopause, then that is something to be aware of. One in a hundred women will enter menopause under the age of 40 years old.

For more on how different perimenopause symptoms affect different women, see Chapter 3.

Let's change the conversation

It's true that knowledge is power – but simply *knowing* how it all works might not necessarily make you *feel* better. If the word 'menopause' makes women in their late 40s and 50s feel old before their time, then 'perimenopause' can be a crushing blow to an even younger woman.

For a variety of reasons, women can be reluctant to confront what's actually happening, but it would be remiss of us not to discuss the ways in which we can be our own worst enemies; denying we're perimenopausal even when the symptoms say otherwise. We're not here to name or shame; we're here to arm and inform you. It's important we get to grips with why we're so hesitant to accept that we're entering perimenopause, so we can move from denial and self-sabotage to empowerment.

So why *do* we feel this way? A lot of the time society paints a picture of menopausal women as grey, not sexy and past their sell-by date. Subliminally, we take in this message that menopause is something for old ladies and we know one thing for certain: we don't want it to be us. In some cultures, fertility dictates a woman's value. If she can no longer have children, does that mean she's past it? Worthless?

The answer is obviously not, but that doesn't dissolve hundreds of years of stigma and negative connotations, so much so that we sometimes hear women wish their symptoms could mean something – anything – else. They say, 'My blood tests are normal, so it can't be my hormones.' It's almost as if they *want* to be anaemic or have an underactive thyroid, or any other tangible, treatable thing they can peg their search for answers on.

This is completely understandable. Coming to the end of your reproductive life can feel like bereavement, even if you never wanted children or are happy with the family you have. Realising you no longer have the choice is tough. But try not to be an ostrich about it. Once you start listening to your body, getting in tune with it, being honest about what's going on, you'll feel lighter. If things don't feel right, don't accept it or deny it, just start finding out more. Repeat after us: your worth is not tied to your ovarian reserves. An exciting new chapter of your life still awaits.

You have the power

Here's the key: although perimenopause is a natural process, you do not have to put up with everything it throws at you. By understanding the changes and being aware of your symptoms, you can make positive lifestyle adjustments and optimise your experience of this time in your life. Our message is: take control of your perimenopause; don't let it take control of you.

We have both heard horror stories about male and female doctors telling patients, 'Well, it's a natural process, what do you want me to do about it?' or 'I don't understand what you're complaining about,' while others take the view that 'it happens to all women, why medicalise it?'

The thing to understand is this: 75 per cent of women experience perimenopausal symptoms that diminish their quality of life, but these symptoms can be treated. We don't buy the idea that women must 'endure' pain or discomfort. When someone has an underactive thyroid, they get thyroid hormone replacement medication. If you were diagnosed with an underactive pancreas in the form of type one diabetes, you would be prescribed the hormone insulin. But if a woman has underactive ovaries, she simply has to suffer? No way. One hundred years ago, we'd be dead by the time we were 60, but now we live until we're 90. Ensuring the second half of our lives is primed for health and happiness isn't something women should be stigmatised for.

In some corners of the medical profession, there's an attitude that sounds something like: 'Every other woman throughout history has put up with it, so why can't you?' But our response is: you don't have to, so why *should* you? We are *not* our mothers or our grandmothers. Our perspective should shift with the times. We parent, work and live in a different way. So why are we still behaving in the same way when it comes to our health?

So, for what might be the first time ever, it's time to make a checklist and put yourself at the top. Our perimenopause motto is #MeFirst. Proactivity is key – and because you have this book in your hands, you've already taken a huge step in the right direction. Now is the time to take charge of your life and put things in order for the decades to come. In all likelihood, you'll find it liberating. We see it as a process of decluttering, re-evaluating and reorganising. Of course, we aren't all the same, but if you spent your 20s trying to build a career and your 30s thinking about your family, it's our philosophy that your 40s and beyond are for prioritising your health and wellbeing so you can get the most out of the next 40 years.

Making medical, lifestyle and emotional changes can seem an overwhelming undertaking at first but, over the course of this book, we're going to break it down and help you be the woman you want to be and feel the way you want to, because how you *feel* is actually more important than anything else. Your inner confidence, your spark, doesn't have to fade away; it can be bright – and shine even brighter. In fact, many women make big professional, sexual and emotional changes at this point in their lives and go on to gain an incredible sense of freedom. Whereas before, you may not have spoken out so much, a lot of women find this is the time they can begin to speak their minds, and really become the woman they want to be without the baggage of other people's expectations.

Yes, navigating perimenopause can be challenging. We're not going to get everything right in one fell swoop and there will be bumps along the road. But when you're armed with information, tools and inspiration, those hiccups will feel more manageable and you'll be able to look forward to feeling empowered for the years to come. So let's get started …

The bottom line

» Recognising you're in perimenopause is the first step towards feeling like yourself again.

» Know your definitions: perimenopause is actually the stage where women experience most of the symptoms they think of as 'menopausal'. Menopause is actually only a one-day event.

» You can make a difference; it's time to listen to your body.

» There's no single type of perimenopause: your set of symptoms will look different to other women's, but they're no less valid.

» See perimenopause in a positive light: there's no need to subscribe to the stigma that so often prevails around women in midlife.

» Use your perimenopause to your advantage as a catalyst for change.

» The power is in your hands: you can be the woman you want to be.

» We want you to use this book to guide you in your perimenopause, so that you are armed with the understanding, knowledge and tools for a good perimenopause.

» Now is the time to take charge. Why not start by filling in the symptoms questionnaire (see page 287) if you haven't yet?

CHAPTER 2

So Much More Than a Hot Flush

Knowledge is power. Being prepared and aware of the symptoms of perimenopause is half the battle.

For most people, 'menopause' and 'hot flushes' go together like strawberries and cream. Those moments of intense heat are what characterise this time in a woman's life because that's how menopause is represented in films, television and magazines. But the full range of perimenopausal symptoms is vast and nuanced, so in this chapter we will decode some of the physical and emotional effects you may be experiencing and cover the full array of symptoms.

Symptoms of perimenopause (see the questionnaire on page 287 to log yours) can creep in over time, and you may not even notice them at first. Your menstrual cycle might shorten by a day or two. You might find yourself getting hot – when in fact it's cold outside. Maybe sleep has been eluding you, but you've put it down to having a lot going on.

With so many symptoms, it's common to find yourself stuck in a vortex of overlapping causes and effects – a chicken-and-egg situation, if you will. You're not sleeping like you used, so you feel tired, so your brain doesn't feel as sharp, so you're forgetful and, as for sex, you have no energy to even think about that! The tiniest symptoms can create confusion. It reminds us of the Dalai Lama's famous aphorism: 'If you think you are too small to make a difference, try sleeping with a mosquito.' Well, if you think a minute shift in hormones is too small to make a difference, try being a perimenopausal woman.

The average age of menopause (when you actually have your last period) is 51, and while some women can sail through perimenopause without any symptoms, three out of four women experience some symptoms from four to ten years before.

Nonetheless, due to a lack of public information and sensitivity around the subject of perimenopause, you may end up self-diagnosing a condition, or putting how you feel down to being a bit knackered and the stresses of being a woman with a busy life, juggling home, work and family. Today's perimenopausal women are often called the 'sand-wich generation' – midlifers whose care responsibilities extend to both their offspring and their elderly parents. They're also the first generation of women who've pursued careers with the same voracity as men, with many starting in the 1980s and 1990s and now holding senior positions. This combination of factors creates a perfect storm that distracts us from what's really going on: perimenopause.

Essentially, when you first start experiencing perimeno-pausal symptoms, you might find it difficult to put your finger on what's happening.

Shereen's story

I went to the hairdresser's for my regular appointment. I'd been going there for years. They tied the cape around my shoulders as normal. Soon after, I felt beads of sweat prickle on my back and run down my spine. I felt paralysed – there was nothing I could do. When I took off the cape, instead of feeling buoyant at my new haircut, I was mortified by the sweat patches that covered my top. I couldn't get out of there quick enough and felt too embarrassed to return.

A symptom as simple as a hot flush can have a crippling effect on a woman's self-esteem and confidence. You might recognise yourself in Shereen's story, and remember how embarrassed and hopeless you felt in the throes of your first few flushes.

Hot flushes are just the tip of the iceberg when it comes to the full spectrum of perimenopausal symptoms. Our narrow understanding of this biologically transformative time in a woman's life is ridden with stereotypes, misinformation and knowledge gaps, meaning that of the 34-plus recognised symptoms, only about five – hot flushes, night sweats, irritability, moodiness and weight gain – are openly discussed. Most women are unaware of the psychological and mood-based perimenopause symptoms that leave them feeling overwhelmed, tired, forgetful and lacking in mental sharpness.

It's time to get acquainted with those symptoms of perimenopause because, after all, knowledge is power.

Key symptoms

This list of symptoms might seem as random as a lucky dip, but if we dig a little deeper, there are common themes.

Headaches

Hair loss

Mood swings

Fatigue

Anxiety

Dizzy spells

Disrupted sleep

Memory lapses

Difficulty concentrating

Depression

Feeling overwhelmed

Panic disorder

Irritability

Hypersensitivity

Burning mouth

Gum soreness

Breast soreness

Irregular heartbeat

Osteoporosis

Hot flushes

Night sweats

Itchy skin

Electric shocks

Weight gain

Allergies/ hives

Hayfever

Body odour

Bloating

Digestive problems

Irregular periods

Vaginal dryness/ itching/burning

Decreased libido

Stress incontinence

Tingling extremities

Brittle nails

Joint pain

Muscle tension

PERIMENOPAUSE SYMPTOMS

We've divided them into eight broad categories: periods, heat, sleep, mental health, physical, digestion, allergies and vaginal health and sex. These categories don't encompass all of the symptoms, but they offer a good framework for examining the key symptoms reported by women in perimenopause.

Periods

Irregular periods are one of the most common symptoms of perimenopause, but they also present a catch-22 situation: the absence of a change to the menstrual cycle can lead some women to believe that they're not perimenopausal, even when they're experiencing many other symptoms. Nonetheless, it's important to give this symptom the prominence it deserves.

Usually, a woman's menstrual cycle begins to get a little shorter – from 30 days to 26, for example. She might not pick up on this subtle shift at first, only noticing when she has two periods in the space of a month – one at the beginning, and one at the end. That, or her partner might say: 'You always seem to be on your period.' After that, periods tend to become more erratic – significantly heavier, lighter or even longer.

Heat

Hot flushes and night sweats are some of the better-known symptoms of perimenopause. They are medically referred to as vasomotor symptoms (VMS).

During a hot flush, the hypothalamus (your body's thermostat) thinks your body is too warm and tries to rid it of heat, causing your blood vessels to dilate. Most women describe the sensation as a creeping feeling of intense heat that spreads across the skin and lasts for several minutes. A hot flush can feel really intense and make the skin redden.

You may feel anxious or panicky and need to go outside, turn on a fan or splash yourself with cold water or use a cooling spray. If you get night sweats, you may have to change your bedding and clothing much more.

Sleep

Changes in sleep can be the tipping point, prompting women to realise their hormones are changing, particularly if they have always enjoyed good sleep. Disrupted sleep – insomnia – can start in early perimenopause and is initially caused by declining progesterone levels and the calming effects they usually bring. Oestrogen decline affects thermoregulation, causing hot flushes and an increase in core body temperature, which is not conducive to a good night's sleep. This disrupts the circadian rhythm, and the increase in body temperature reduces levels of melatonin (see page 139), the hormone responsible for our sleep–wake cycle. So, all these factors mean we end up with less of our deepest non-REM stage 3 sleep, which leaves us feeling tired and often hungry the next day. Women who've enjoyed good sleep throughout their lives are affected so much so that the hours between 3am and 5am are often referred to as the perimenopause 'waking hours'.

Mental health

You won't have failed to notice that several of the symptoms (see page 23) are related to emotional wellbeing – and even those that aren't directly connected, such as bloating, muscle tension, headaches and itchy skin, can be indirectly caused by stress.

During perimenopause, our coping skills feel depleted and this lack of resilience causes some women to experience mental health issues for what might be the first time ever. If you're struggling with symptoms that are ostensibly connected to sleep and heat, for example, you might find the stress of these affects your mood too.

Highlighting the psychological symptoms is important because they're the ones that are harder to put your finger on and also to get a doctor to take seriously and equate to your hormones. But you're not going crazy – they are real symptoms. Ovarian function is closely related to brain function because we have oestrogen receptors in our brain. In many ways oestrogen is like the brain's Wi-Fi; it helps connectivity. Oestrogen increases the production of sero-tonin, dopamine and noradrenaline – the happy chemicals – in the brain, and has an impact on the brain's nerve function. When our oestrogen is dipping, our brain feels slower, and we become frustrated with ourselves because of it. If you often forget what you are about to say and have frustrating 'tip-of-the-tongue' moments, the perimenopause might be why. You may even worry that you are getting early Alzheim-er's or dementia, which can be anxiety-provoking in itself.

Yet why is it you don't feel like this every day? It's because your mental and emotional symptoms will fluctu-ate alongside your oestrogen levels. Mood swings, anxiety, memory lapses, fatigue, difficulty concentrating, irritability, depression and panic disorder are all symptoms we see as the basic ways in which perimenopause may impact mental health, but you might experience many more emotions that come up as a result of hormonal changes related to peri-menopause. Feel indecisive, flat, foggy and blunted? They're not on the official list, but they're real and they're symp-toms a significant number of women experience.

Physical

It might seem vain to worry about changes to your weight, skin and hair, but these might be indicators of perimenopause and we shouldn't shame women for talking about them.

Similarly, itchy skin, hair loss and brittle nails are all symptoms of perimenopause – oestrogen is an essential ingredient for stimulating collagen, elastin and hyaluronic acid production, all of which are essential for maintaining healthy, shiny hair and skin. From the age of 25, we lose 1 per cent of collagen per year, and this significantly accelerates to 30 per cent loss in the first five years post-menopause, causing us to look older and the skin on our face to become less elastic and sag, giving rise to jowls, and giving some women the appearance of looking angry or frowning all the time. Also hormonal changes cause dryness, creating flakey, less plump skin all over our bodies, not forgetting our vulva and vagina because we have collagen there too.

Women also complain of weight gain during perimenopause – and it's 100 per cent a legitimate complaint. It's down to a combination of less movement, a slower metabolism and changes to insulin sensitivity (see page 162), which increases fat stores, particularly around the middle. Weight gain has a huge impact on self-esteem and there are associated health risks, such as diabetes, so now is the time to make changes (see Chapter 15).

The physical symptoms of perimenopause include various aches and pains, including headaches (and in extreme cases, migraines – see page 197), breast soreness, joint pain and muscle tension. Oestrogen reduces inflammation between joints, so having less or fluctuating levels of it will cause joint pain. Similarly, declining oestrogen levels cause breast pain and breast tissue shrinks as the body realises it no longer needs its milk-making system, so you may notice sagging.

Digestion

Hormonal changes in perimenopause affect our gut and slow down digestion. Bloating is a common symptom caused by the hormonal shifts and you may have more gas, constipation, irregular bowel movements and nausea (see Chapter 12).

Allergies

There's also a link between perimenopause and allergies. Our bodies become more sensitive and are less able to process histamine, which our bodies release as a natural immune response to inflammation, so you may find that symptoms such as hay fever, asthma and prickly heat rash get worse during this time. For a deeper dive into histamine intolerance, go to page 208.

Vaginal health and sex

Changes to hormone levels often cause a loss of libido as well as urinary symptoms. This is known as genitourinary syndrome of menopause (GSM) as it encompasses vaginal, urinary and pelvic floor issues that affect women due to menopause. So just because you're having periods doesn't mean your fluctuating hormone levels aren't impacting your overall vaginal health.

To explain what's happening inside the vagina of a woman in perimenopause, think back to your school science lessons. Our normal vaginal pH is 3.4 to 4.5 – acidic on litmus paper, which would show as orange. But during perimenopause, the drop in oestrogen causes our vagina to become more alkaline blue on the litmus paper.

This shift from acidic to alkaline has consequences. Acid is a protective barrier and prevents bacteria coming into our vagina. As the pH changes, the walls of the vagina become thin and crepe-like and externally the vulva also loses some of its plumpness, making you more prone to getting infections like thrush and cystitis. We also lose some of our natural lubrication, which can make sex really uncomfortable and adds to the loss of libido (see Chapter 7).

We can't talk about vaginal health without discussing what perimenopause does to our pelvic floor, the 'hammock' of muscles that extends from the bottom to the front of the pubic bone and supports the pelvic organs, including the bladder, bowel and womb. If you leak when you cough or sneeze, you'll know just how important the pelvic floor is. In fact, we've met women who refuse to wear pale trousers or skirts for fear of leaking.

In our younger years, these muscles are springy and supportive, but as oestrogen levels change, so too does the effectiveness of the pelvic floor. Pelvic floor exercises help, but they won't compensate for the lack of oestrogen, which means you won't get the pelvic floor's support back without some extra oestrogen. Even if you're not keen on hormone replacement therapy (see Chapter 4), a course of 'localised' oestrogen (which take the form of a pessary, cream or vaginal ring) can really help with vaginal and pelvic floor symptoms. The dose is incredibly low – localised oestrogen over a year is equivalent to one to two day's worth of systemic HRT, so if your symptoms are particularly localised and you find yourself worrying about leaks and panty liners, that's something to consider.

Tracking your symptoms

It might take time for your doctor to make the connection between your symptoms and perimenopause, so it's worth writing them down. You could use a period-tracking app, such as Period Tracker or Clue, and record when you've had a hot flush, a bad night's sleep or are just feeling more irritable than usual. It won't help to become obsessive about it, but knowing what happens when will make you more confident when talking to your doctor and help you be kinder to yourself when you know you're likely to experience trickier symptoms.

Not all symptoms are equally likely to appear throughout your entire perimenopause; some are characteristic of early perimenopause, whereas others tend to occur later. This diagram shows which symptoms to expect at each stage, and where there might be some overlap.

Long-term symptoms

Often women think that when their periods stop, so will their symptoms, but they can also persist after your last period (menopause) and well into post-menopause.

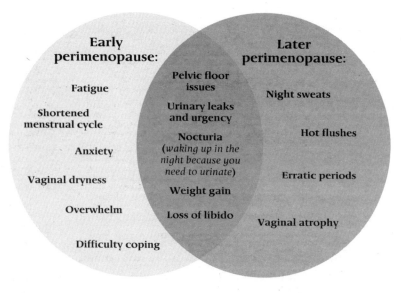

EARLY VS LATER SYMPTOMS

What we haven't discussed yet – and doesn't get so much airtime in the mainstream media and in conversations around menopause – are the long-term health conditions that women are at higher risk of. Being prepared and being aware can help you minimise the risk.

Dementia: twice as many women suffer from dementia than men post-menopause. Though the reason for this is not fully understood, we know oestrogen and testosterone play a role in maintaining and protecting the brain and that brain function can decline by 30 per cent post-menopause. One of the reasons why men are 'protected' is because they maintain their testosterone levels throughout their lives, retaining the protective effect.

Diabetes: women in this stage of their lives will often see their levels of bad cholesterol (LDL, non-HDL) rise, as well as triglycerides (a type of fat), putting them at a higher risk of Type 2 diabetes.

Osteoporosis: this is a condition whereby the bones become more fragile due to reduced bone mass and bone deterioration, a consequence of hormonal loss post-menopause. One in three women over 50 and one in five men over 50 end up having a fracture due to this. You can protect against it through diet (see page 205) and weight-bearing exercise (see page 238).

Cardiovascular disease: women lose the protective effect of the hormone oestrogen post-menopause, making it the biggest cause of death of women worldwide – five times more so than breast cancer.

Depression: men still account for three-quarters of suicides in the UK but, in women, the highest rate is among those aged 45–49 – again right in the middle of perimenopause.

... And if you've gone through an earlier menopause or have a family history of any of these conditions, then your risks are greater. The loss of the protective effects of oestrogen is the main culprit, but many women aren't aware. Their concerns are the things impacting them in the here and now, such as not being able to sleep, weight gain and mood swings. They want to know how to deal with the present, not what they might be at higher risk of when they're 70. And we get it: when you can't sleep through the night or make it an hour without sweating through your clothes, life can become about simply getting through the next few weeks, months and not years.

Addressing your symptoms

The good news is that you don't have to stoically plod on – something we've found British women to be spectacularly good at!

Helen's story

My friend recommended that I make an appointment with Dr Harper after seeing me have a hot flush. I wasn't a menopause denier, per se, but I was pretty reluctant to engage with the idea that I might be changing. In general, my mood, relationship, my life was fine – well, that's what I thought.

At the appointment we discussed my diet, and Dr Harper advised me to take more regular exercise, cut back on the G&Ts and 'chill out' more – she recommended mindfulness. I was prescribed the hormone treatment Oestrogel to help with the hot flushes. I'd had a hysterectomy so I didn't need any progesterone hormone.

Ten weeks later, we did a review via Zoom and my husband joined the call. He wanted to thank Dr Harper for the difference the medication had made to my life and his. All this time, I hadn't known how much better I could have felt. I'd been putting up with the symptoms for so long – losing my sense of fun and being constantly snappy and irritable had become my new normal. I was still doing all the same things, but I hadn't realised how much effort it was taking. Without knowing it, I was exhausted from the effort of maintaining the life I'd always lived, but HRT made me feel like myself again.

Helen's story is typical of the kind we hear all the time: women who are so determined to be themselves they don't realise how much effort they're putting into making every-thing appear normal. Because the symptoms happen slowly and take time to develop, they compensate gradually and don't realise just how much of themselves they're losing.

The symptoms of perimenopause can be overwhelm-ing and – at times – downright scary, but with the right approach, it can be a productive, empowering time. Many women start new relationships or businesses at this age and stage.

You'll feel your very best if you address your symptoms early on. Don't think of proactivity as a burden, but a golden ticket to a liberating second wind. Some prominent voices in the menopause conversation talk of 'feeling amazing when you're out the other side' or 'being able to step into the most fearless version of yourself once "The Change" is over'. Words like these might give you the impression peri-menopause is something to endure. Let us clue you into a secret: it's not. Let's change that narrative and instead think of it as a positive reset and rebalance.

We want you to be the best you can be right *now*. Don't wait. You can start by filling out the symptom checklist (see page 287), if you haven't yet, and taking it to your doctor.

The bottom line

» Don't pass off your symptoms as 'life': if you're in your 40s and things feel strange, you might be in perimenopause.
» Be informed: familiarise yourself with the wide range of perimenopausal symptoms (see page 23). They range from electric shocks to hair loss – not just hot flushes.
» Localised oestrogen for vulvo-vaginal health can be a game-changer and is safe for most women.
» Think long-term: perimenopause and menopause leave women at higher risk of conditions like dementia and osteoporosis later in life.
» Don't resign yourself to battling through because of media horror stories: help is always available. Empower yourself!

CHAPTER 3

No Two Journeys Are The Same

Hearing menopause discussed by a wide spectrum of voices with different perspectives is important because we all experience it differently.

There is no one-size-fits-all, fixed 'route' to menopause, but there is a core narrative that dictates what perimenopause and menopause are. In this chapter, we'll look at what perimenopause and its corresponding symptoms can look like for a range of diverse and different women so that you don't feel alone in this identity-shifting time of your life.

Approximately three-quarters of women will get perimenopausal symptoms and, for some, they can be severely detrimental to their wellbeing and quality of life. Similarly, the perimenopausal journey can be short and sweet for some and long and protracted for others.

There are, of course, common threads and you might find when you mention a symptom while having coffee with friends, it often serves as a catalyst for everyone to chime in with the same or similar symptoms, like opening a peri-menopausal Pandora's Box. These moments can feel like a huge relief, but every woman is unique and, despite the commonalities, none of us will go through the same experience; even if we have the same symptoms, we all experience things differently because of who we are.

It's also about how we respond to those symptoms. You personally might be able to handle the hot flushes, but find that the loss of mental clarity and sharpness is what most impacts *your* quality of life. Someone else might really struggle with night sweats and sleep disturbance. For a woman in a new relationship, the loss of libido, vaginal dryness, and skin and hair changes may be her greatest concern. We each have our own tipping point and trigger to go to see the doctor.

Premature menopause

One of the ways a woman's experience might veer from the 'norm' is if she goes through perimenopause before she was expecting to and before her friends. This can be a shock and may leave her feeling bereft and less feminine. The average age of menopause is 51, but 5 per cent of women go through a natural 'early menopause' between the ages of 40 and 45. A further 1 per cent will go through menopause before they reach 40, and this is categorised as primary ovarian insufficiency (POI), or premature menopause. One in 1,000 women will go through menopause, i.e. have their last period, under the age of 30, and one in 10,000, under the age of 20.

POI is diagnosed if your menopause occurs before the age of 40. It can be caused by a genetic disease, such as Turner syndrome, and some autoimmune conditions, such as Hashimoto's disease and Graves' disease (when the immune system mistakenly attacks the thyroid gland). Stress can also accelerate the process of hormonal decline, which means a traumatic event, like the loss of a parent or loved one, can be a cause or contributing factor. Lifestyle elements like smoking, poor diet and lack of exercise, as well as IVF treatment (see page 44), can also contribute to an earlier menopause. There are many things that can trigger POI and – frustratingly – it won't always be possible to determine the exact cause. This grey area can make women feel angry and confused.

Sara's story

I'm 34 and six years ago I realised my periods had become less regular; in fact, I'd missed a couple but put it down to the fact that I had started going running a lot. It didn't enter my mind for a second that I could be perimenopausal.

Nonetheless, something niggled at me and I wanted to rule out anything serious, so I went to see my doctor, who told me to come back in three months if my periods still hadn't returned to normal and in the meantime to stop running and gain some weight. This made no difference, so at my next appointment I had a blood test. The results showed I had a raised FSH level, and I was diagnosed with POI.

I'd always wanted to have children, so this diagnosis was nothing short of devastating. What compounded my pain was that I was given virtually no information or advice, and was just put on the contraceptive pill. At no point did anyone explain the increased risks of osteoporosis and cardiovascular disease, or the risk to my psychological and mental health and wellbeing.

The internet has been a great source of information as has social media. I've discovered support groups and, in particular, The Daisy Network who also help women like me to become mothers through adoption or egg donation, which I am considering. I don't feel so alone and I've decided to change to body-identical HRT (see page 59) rather than the contraceptive pill as it feels more natural to me. I'm definitely now in a better headspace than I was a couple of years ago.

Surgical and medical menopause

Early or premature menopause can also be induced or accelerated by a surgical procedure, or by radiation and chemotherapy for cancer treatment. When this happens, it's known as 'surgical or medical menopause', depending on its cause.

A full hysterectomy (where the womb and ovaries are removed) will cause women to become menopausal overnight. Partial hysterectomies, where the womb is removed but the ovaries are retained, will likely also induce a surgical menopause, but the transition may feel gentler and less sudden because the ovaries continue producing hormones. Many cancer treatments can also affect the ovaries, rendering them inactive.

If you're going to have a medical procedure that's likely to bring on perimenopausal symptoms or even the menopause itself, you should be fully counselled and made aware of what to expect by a multidisciplinary medical team, including a counsellor. And if your doctor is particularly astute, you may be offered HRT (see Chapter 4) straight away post-recovery, if appropriate.

The symptoms of an early or premature perimenopause are the same as those that occur at the average age, but certain symptoms, e.g. loss of fertility, loss of libido, vaginal atrophy and ageing, can have a greater impact on a woman's self-confidence, self-esteem and mental health. Women who have gone through an earlier menopause are at a higher risk of depression. Medical hormone replacement treatment is important for those women who have gone through an early or premature menopause. Oestrogen – as we know – is paramount, and progesterone is still needed for women who have gone through early menopause (unless your perimenopausal symptoms were surgically induced due to a hysterectomy). In both instances, testosterone (see page 54) is also a key player – especially for younger women – as it helps maintain energy, muscle mass, libido and mental sharpness. Sometimes younger women are offered the contraceptive pill, like Sara was (see page 37), rather than HRT because of wanting to fit in with their friends and not 'feel old'. The combined pill contains both oestrogen and progesterone, so can also do the job of helping the women to feel 'normal'.

All younger women should be on some form of hormone replacement treatment, at least until the average age of menopause, to reduce their long-term health risks and keep their hormone levels in line with the general female population. Oestrogen protects blood vessels and the heart, as well as being important for maintaining bone density and strength. For these reasons, someone going through an early menopause should have regular check-ups and DEXA scans to monitor bone density as osteoporosis (see page 31) is one of the major downsides of decreased oestrogen production.

Alongside hormonal treatment, women going through early or premature menopause may need emotional or psychological support through counselling and support groups, which may be accessed from their doctor, online or directly via the NHS. The lack of oestrogen gives rise to menopausal mood disturbances, which can cause low mood, anxiety, loss of confidence and brain fog. But, moreover, the sense of loss many women experience with an early menopause can be like a reactive depression, and can even – in some cases – extend to clinical depression. Many women find they have a combination of both. In these instances, do seek help, speak to your doctor who can refer you for counselling, such as cognitive behavioural therapy (CBT), and offer antidepressant medication, which can all help.

Lifestyle, cultural and medical factors

Recently, we were in a taxi when the driver asked us what we do for a living. We told him we were healthcare professionals specialising in menopause. If we're honest, we were both expecting his eyes to shift away from his mirror and for an awkward silence to engulf us for the rest of the trip. Instead, he didn't flinch, and told us – in sympathetic tones – all about his wife, who'd just been through menopause. He said there should be more help for women as he had seen how his wife had lost all her confidence and there should be more information and education for partners, so they knew how to be supportive, and he's absolutely right. There's more on how to talk to partners and children about perimenopause in Chapter 6.

As our taxi ride proves, as a society we're becoming more comfortable discussing menopause, in public and in private. As more high-profile women are beginning to talk openly about their experience of perimenopause, so the stigma declines. There's no doubt raising awareness in this way will help thousands of women understand their symptoms and, frankly, feel less like they're going insane. We believe that any conversation that shines a light on perimenopause and menopause is a good thing.

Diversity makes the world go round

We need to be more inclusive when we're talking about menopause because half of the world's population goes through it. I'm sure we weren't the only ones to do a happy dance when Michelle Obama talked about her experience in her podcast, because it's so rare to hear Black women – and women of colour generally – talk about it.

When the former editor of *Vogue*, Alexandra Shulman, discussed her experience of the menopause in a column for the *Daily Mail*, there was initial delight because, again, more conversation is great. But she went on to say that she believes we should stop 'banging on' about menopausal symptoms, and that's where we disagree. She admitted that she hadn't suffered 'debilitating symptoms', that she took HRT and retired from a well-paid job with a corporate pension. But there are a lot of women who aren't as fortunate. For them, more understanding and conversation around menopause could mean more access to care and treatment, which could be life-changing in terms of continuing in their jobs and, in some cases, salvaging relationships.

Hearing menopause discussed by a wide spectrum of voices with different perspectives is important because we all experience it differently. If a dominant narrative emerges based on what's most commonly discussed by one type of woman, it can create confusion among those whose experience is different.

There are a number of cultural and lifestyle factors that will affect how we all experience menopause, which are explained below.

What we eat

The Western diet often contains more processed foods, refined sugars and saturated fat because of cheaper, easier fast-food options. In the West, rates of obesity are higher and, thanks to the insulin dysregulation associated with takeaways and fast foods, vasomotor symptoms like hot sweats, night sweats and hot flushes are more prevalent. Relatively high alcohol and caffeine consumption in Western diets worsens these vasomotor symptoms and makes us more prone to heart palpitations and anxiety.

Research has shown that for Southeast Asian women, aches, pains and fatigue dominate, rather than hot flushes – perhaps because alcohol isn't so widely consumed. In these countries, pelvic issues, stress incontinence, vaginal dryness and atrophy can be more common, causing more frequent urinary tract infections and thrush. Whereas Japanese women who have a diet high in soy (plant oestrogen) have fewer vasomotor symptoms and experience headaches, shoulder stiffness and chilliness. Filipino women have more headaches and Lebanese women often present with fatigue and irritability.

Working out

We often hear women with perimenopausal symptoms say they're worried about exercising because it makes them sweat more and causes hot flushes, so they avoid it altogether. But, actually, exercising reduces stress levels, increases the release of endorphins and the happy hormones (serotonin, noradrenaline and dopamine), maintains and builds muscle strength, enhances brain clarity and function, and helps with metabolism and overall weight. That's quite a list, but the benefits really are endless (see Chapter 13). Women who exercise regularly also find they can manage their symptoms better, have a more positive mental attitude and are less overweight. Remember, working out is about doing something you enjoy, not running on a treadmill until your legs feel like jelly.

How we live

If you're someone who thrives on adrenaline and has a lifestyle to match, you'll likely have more perimenopausal symptoms than someone who lives in a less high-octane way. Cortisol is the stress hormone, and raised levels – which you'll have if you're a thrill-seeker with a lot of stress – will likely mean you have more symptoms of greater severity. It's for this reason that working women living in busy cities have more symptoms compared to women who don't work and live in the countryside.

Whether or not we work and how many hours we work will have an impact on the extent of our symptoms: when women say, 'But my mother didn't have any symptoms', it might simply be because she hid them, but it might also be because she didn't have to deal with the stress of juggling a demanding, 40-plus-hours-per-week job alongside raising children, as so many women do today. Women's lives are far more stressful now than they were 20 years ago.

Our education

It's a sad fact that women who are less affluent, in lower socioeconomic groups, have a harder time going through perimenopausal symptoms than their richer counterparts – for a variety of reasons, including a poorer-quality diet and higher rates of smoking and obesity. Levels of education also play a role in our menopausal journeys: a lack of education may mean a woman suffers unnecessarily because she doesn't know her treatment options or understand her symptoms. Having an increased awareness and understanding can be the difference between surviving, thriving and soaring through perimenopause.

Parenthood and relationships

Whether you've given birth or not, and how you came to conceive, will also have an impact on your experience of perimenopause. Women who've not had children or had them under the age of 28 years often go through an earlier perimenopause and menopause. Women who have gone through IVF cycles tend to find they experience perimenopausal symptoms and menopause sooner as their ovaries have been hyperstimulated by hormones, accelerating the journey to perimenopause.

If you've had children, especially by vaginal delivery, then you'll be more likely to experience pelvic floor problems, such as leaking when sneezing or coughing, and even when exercising, due to the strain on the pelvic floor muscles during pregnancy.

Your medical background

Though you may not have had the kinds of surgeries or treatments that can bring on early menopause (see page 36), your individual medical history and body mass index (BMI) might affect your perimenopause experience. Very underweight women can enter menopause earlier because in order to function their bodies switch off ovarian hormonal activity. They also have lower body fat, and body fat also produces a weak form of oestrogen. So, the combination of these two factors initiates an earlier perimenopause due to the overall reduction in oestrogen, increasing the risk of osteoporosis. (Note that one of the reasons we gain midriff fat in midlife is because our body is trying to compensate for the decline of oestrogen production from our ovaries, so it tries to produce some from fat.) Conversely, women who are overweight or obese tend to go through menopause later, because they have longer exposure to oestrogen which increases their risk of ovarian and womb cancer.

If you have polycystic ovarian syndrome (PCOS), you may actually find – ironically – some of your PCOS symptoms improve as your perimenopausal symptoms ramp up. Irregular periods, a common symptom of PCOS, can either become more irregular or may, funnily enough, during perimenopause become *more* regular because hormonal fluctuations cancel each other out. Confusing, I know!

A similar thing can happen if you have an underactive thyroid (hypothyroidism), as this causes heavy periods, fatigue and weight gain. An overactive thyroid (hyperthyroidism) can cause palpitations, missed periods, anxiety and chronic fatigue syndrome; the symptoms of perimenopause and those conditions can mimic each other, causing doubt and uncertainty about what's really going on. If you have chronic fatigue syndrome and you're feeling more wiped out than ever, don't dismiss it – you might be in perimenopause.

Medical conditions that can mimic perimenopause

» Anaemia: iron deficiency, vitamin B12 deficiency
» Vitamin D deficiency
» Underactive thyroid
» Overactive thyroid
» Chronic fatigue syndrome
» Fibromyalgia
» Depression
» Long Covid

Contraception

Hormonal contraception can mask your 'natural' hormone levels and therefore your understanding of what's going on in your body.

Technically you can safely stay on the combined oral contraceptive pill until the age of 50, so long as you are fit and healthy, but because it contains oestrogen and a form of progesterone it may mask perimenopausal symptoms. If you're a smoker, or have high blood pressure or diabetes, then your doctor will often suggest switching to a progesterone-only pill at around aged 40 to reduce your risk of blood clots, which can cause strokes and heart disease.

Once you've made the switch, your body will regulate and rebalance itself and, without the addition of oestrogen, you'll fairly quickly start to get the perimenopausal symptoms your friends might have been experiencing for a while: joint pains, hot flushes, vaginal dryness, broken sleep – by now you know the drill. Suddenly, your smear test might feel a bit uncomfortable, or sex might require a little more lube.

The progesterone-only contraception stops the menstrual cycle for 70 per cent of women. This means you won't know if your cycle has become shorter or more irregular, so it is important not to look to your cycle for confirmation as to whether or not you're perimenopausal. Go by how you feel.

The same goes for women on other forms of progesterone-only contraceptives, such as the implant and the Mirena coil (a hormonal intrauterine device containing progesterone). The Mirena coil is commonly used as a contraceptive for women in their 40s as it also helps to reduce heavy periods and completely stops them in 50–70 per cent of women. If you had the Mirena coil fitted for this reason, it could now be masking the fact that your heavy periods were a sign of the perimenopause. It's important to think about what other symptoms you may have been experiencing.

Women with the Mirena coil may benefit from having a blood test to measure their FSH levels, as it may indicate whether or not they are in perimenopause. That said, the caveat is that because hormone levels can fluctuate during perimenopause, a blood test might still show normal FSH levels and require a further test six weeks later.

Hina's story

At aged 48, I'd started to experience symptoms of fatigue and irritability, snapping at the smallest of things. I was also finding it difficult to sleep and was starting to wonder if I was perimenopausal. Eighteen months earlier, I'd had the Mirena coil fitted and hadn't had a period since, so I had no idea what my 'natural' cycle was doing. I was advised to have a blood test to check my FSH level as the coil and lack of menstrual cycle could be masking my menopause.

I had a raised FSH of 43, and my oestrogen levels were low – no wonder I was feeling rubbish (a FSH of 25 is an indicator of menopause). It was the jolt I needed to overhaul my life. I had 'let myself go' – my weight had been creeping up and due to the pressures of work had forgotten to take time out for myself. I started to diarise half an hour each day to go for a walk, which then became a jog. Also, I started to keep a food diary to track how much I was actually eating. I realised that I had started drinking more, which was adding unnecessary calories and making me feel bloated. My memory was still something that was worrying me, so I decided to try hormone therapy and was prescribed oestrogen gel, which I applied to my upper inner leg. A combination of all these things has started to help me feel more like me again.

Of course, none of us have just one contributing factor – we are middle class Southeast Asian women who smoke and have had no children; we are working class white women who exercise frequently and had IVF; we are Black women who have PCOS and are on the contraceptive pill. We're all a series of intersections, a complex web of factors, each of which will have its own bearing on our unique experience of perimenopause. Many aspects of our lives will overlap in ways that at times seem conflicting and contradictory, and at others seem to make perfect sense. That's why it's useful to have an overview of the different ways in which meno-pause might affect you depending on your lifestyle, culture and medical background – even if that's just to reassure you that you're not going mad, because things really are as confusing as they sound.

Trans menopause

If you're a trans woman, you will most likely have been on a hormone journey that includes prescribed oestrogen, possibly progesterone, plus a testosterone blocker. Perimenopause and meno-pause are almost always framed around cisgender women's experiences – something we hope is changing – but perimenopause-like symptoms may well affect you if your hormones fluctuate or if you have to suddenly stop taking your hormone ther-apy. Hormone therapy is highly individualised so, along with your healthcare provider, you will need to weigh up quality of life and wellbeing, as well as potential long-term risks of any medications you're taking. As always, it's best to seek out advice and guidance from a practitioner well versed in the latest hormone research.

As a trans man it is likely that you will experience perimenopause-type symptoms, which can have short- and long-term effects. If you're using high levels of testosterone, you may well find that your lowering oestrogen levels cause vaginal discomfort (whether or not you've had genital reassignment surgery) and increase the likelihood of UTIs and infections like thrush (see page 28). Long-term risks include losing bone strength and osteoporosis, which both need to be thoroughly considered and guarded against (see Chapter 13). Depending on your personal situation, you might also need to think about breast cancer screening and smear tests.

If you don't feel comfortable talking to your doctor, contact Stonewall (see page 299) for a list of NHS organisations who have signed up to the Diversity Champions programme.

Reaching acceptance

Our personal circumstances will have an impact on how we experience perimenopause through our symptoms, but they'll also dictate how accepting we are of the process.

Different cultures have different levels of acceptance when it comes to the menopause. In many European and American cultures, the female 'ideal' is sexy, attractive and youthful, while ageing is seen as deeply negative. Women who've lived their lives burdened by these stereotypes and expectations are going to find it harder to accept the menopause.

In Southeast Asian cultures, however, ageing is seen as more positive; something that makes you wiser, a leader in your community. In some societies, like Greek Orthodox, where contraception isn't so readily used, it's a liberating time, because it's only once they've reached menopause that women have sexual freedom and don't have to worry about getting pregnant.

Regardless of where you're from, though, acceptance is a personal journey. In our experience when it comes to treating hundreds of perimenopausal women, reaching a place of peace – and then proactivity – is key if you're to allow yourself to truly regain control of your life.

The bottom line

» Your experience of the perimenopause is just that – yours. If you're having different symptoms from your peer group, it doesn't mean you're not in perimenopause, or that your experience is any less valid.

» Beware of media coverage: more talk is great, but coverage often focuses on a narrow set of symptoms (like hot flushes). Look for conversations around perimenopause that include diverse voices.

» Pause for thought and reflect on the factors – diet, exercise habits, medical history, choice of contraception – that influence your symptoms. Make a note of them if that helps.

» Acceptance is a personal journey: some cultures are far more welcoming of midlife women than others and if yours is not one of them, then it's time for us to change the narrative.

CHAPTER 4

Hormone Replacement Therapy

There are some truths and a lot of myths around Hormone Replacement Therapy (HRT), so let's do some demystifying.

HRT is not a panacea or a magic wand; it is not for everyone and some women can't take it for medical reasons. Whether or not to begin taking HRT, also called medical hormone treatment or menopausal hormone therapy (MHT), is still one of the most contentious decisions a woman can make as she navigates perimenopause. So, in this chapter, we take a closer look at the persistent myths around HRT, the many forms it comes in and the risks so you can make an informed choice.

Simone's story

At 47 years old, my periods were still sort of regular, although I had missed the odd few. I'd been feeling flat and irritable for years and had tried virtually every lifestyle measure to mitigate my symptoms: yoga, exercising, taking over-the-counter supplements. I'd become an expert on sage supplements, maca, ashwagandha ... But now I was at the end of my tether – I needed help, but I was adamant I didn't want to take HRT.

I'd once read a newspaper article about the breast cancer risks associated with certain types of HRT, and it had put me off for life. However, after talking through the latest research, the different types of HRT, and gaining some perspective on how the dangers of HRT compared to say, drinking a glass of wine every night (see page 64), I was sold and completely changed my opinion. After a few weeks of being on HRT, I couldn't believe how much better I felt.

Helena's story

At age 53 I almost had to be pushed through the clinic door by a friend. I'd been experiencing debilitating hot flushes, but was being stoic and typically English about it, insisting I was absolutely fine, and flatly denying I needed medication, dismissing it as 'unnecessary'. After discussing the pros and cons of HRT, I decided to go for it. A month later I felt so much calmer. I realised I'd been angry for five years, but hadn't known why.

These two stories (and, trust us, there are *many* more) show the conversation around HRT is riddled with myths, misinformation and preconceptions – some of which you may be mulling over in your own mind and all of which we'll address in this chapter, so get ready for some myth-busting, starting with some common concerns we hear over and over again.

Common concerns

1. 'Will I get breast cancer if I go on HRT?'
    No, not all HRT preparations have the same risks.
2. 'Do I have to wait for my periods to stop before starting HRT?'
    No, you can start HRT during your perimenopause.
3. 'Can I only go on HRT for five years?'
    No, there's no finite time.
4. 'HRT is unnatural, isn't it?'
    There are lots of different preparations, some of which are plant-based and body-identical (see page 59).
5. 'Doesn't taking HRT mean I'm fighting ageing?'
    It is true that menopause is a natural part of ageing, but we can make it an easier journey.
6. 'Will HRT cause weight gain?'
    Not necessarily. There are many reasons for potential weight gain during perimenopause and hormonal imbalance is one of them, so correcting it can actually be beneficial to maintaining a healthy weight.
7. 'Won't I slip back into my symptoms as soon as I come off HRT?'
    Firstly, you don't have to come off it. If you decide to, then do so gradually, tapering down the dose. If you stop suddenly, you may get some 'rebound' symptoms.

What is hormone replacement therapy (HRT)?

HRT is one of those medical terms that very much does what it says on the tin: it's a form of medical hormone treatment to relieve the symptoms of perimenopause and menopause by topping up and replacing the hormones your ovaries are no longer producing. When we refer to HRT, we are commonly referring to oestrogen and progesterone replacement. However, there can be a role for the hormone testosterone too (see page 60).

Let's pause for a moment for a quick history lesson. The scientist Edward Doisy first discovered oestrogen in 1929. In 1942 it was isolated from the urine of pregnant mares and approved, as Premarin, by the FDA for the treatment of hot flushes. This was almost 20 years before the contraceptive pill.

In the 1960s in his book *Feminine Forever*, the gynaecologist Robert A Wilson claimed 'Menopause was a preventable event, because women could simply add back the oestrogen their body was no longer making by taking hormone pills.' Following this, women started seeking hormone treatment from their doctors. Until the mid-70s women were prescribed oestrogen replacement alone. While symptoms may have improved, unfortunately, due to the unopposed oestrogen, the rate of endometrial cancer increased eightfold. Progesterone was needed to counterbalance the oestrogen effects on the womb lining and reduce the risk of endometrial cancers.

A note on testosterone

As testosterone is thought of as 'a male hormone', its role in a woman's physiology is wildly underestimated and misunderstood, yet it's crucial to be aware of how it works in our bodies.

In women, testosterone is produced by the ovaries and adrenal glands, which sit on top of the kidneys. It helps to build muscle mass, bone strength and bone mineral density, maintain our sex drives and libido, and is also part responsible for brain sharpness and focus.

Our testosterone levels decline by approximately 50 per cent between our 20s and 40s (for men it's a gradual decline from their mid-40s onwards), which means the first symptoms of perimenopause – fatigue, lack of energy, lower quality sleep and a reduced libido – are often those caused by decreasing testosterone levels. When women say, 'I've not gained weight, but I've lost muscle tone in the tops of my arms and legs,' they're talking about sarcopenia, the technical term for a loss of muscle mass, which is caused by declining levels of testosterone.

It's important to consider whether making testosterone part of your HRT prescription is right for you (see page 60) – too often it goes ignored, but its effectiveness when it comes to mitigating the above symptoms can be significant.

What's right for you?

The starting point for us is always to take a holistic view and advise women to look first at her 'modifiable lifestyle factors' – the changes she can make to help herself. And then, if needed, safely add HRT. So many women are made to feel like failures for opting for HRT, or not taking the supplement-only route, and we want to change that.

It is true that in perimenopause, especially the early stages, symptoms can often be managed by the diet, lifestyle changes and supplements that we will be discussing in depth in later chapters, but there can often be a tipping point for women when 'more' is needed. What we want to do in this book is to dispel those scare stories, so women who want or need to be on hormone therapy aren't missing out and literally suffering in silence because of misinformation.

We live half our lives in perimenopause and beyond. In perimenopause our ovaries are underactive; they're no longer producing the hormones that supported our bodies in the same way as before. The body is in a hormone-deficient state in the same way it is with an underactive thyroid, and people don't think twice about medicating that condition. Your ovaries are going through a change: they're under-producing hormones, which can affect brain function, heart health, digestion, the skin and hair – causing you to feel less like yourself and increasing the risk of long-term health issues.

If you're worried about if and when to start taking HRT because you see it as putting something unnatural into your body, don't. In the same way that we are all different and have different needs, there are many preparations and formulations, including plant-based and natural, that could be the right fit for you.

When the time is right HRT may help with some of the more immediate symptoms of perimenopause, such as insomnia, night sweats, hot flushes and anxiety. Taken alongside diet and lifestyle changes, it can also reduce your future risk of developing some of the longer-term health issues (see page 30), such as diabetes, heart disease, osteoporosis and dementia.

However, nothing is ever risk-free and we need to bear this in mind when we make our choices (see page 59).

When to start HRT

The changes that occur in a woman's body when she enters perimenopause can, if ignored, increase the risk of cardio-vascular disease, dementia and stroke. That's why the British Heart Foundation advocates attention to your diet (see Part 3) to lower your bad cholesterol. Also, to take regular exercise to maintain your muscle mass (not forgetting your heart is also a muscle that needs a workout) and reducing those factors that increase blood clots, such as smoking and being overweight. If HRT is a consideration, then studies have shown that the optimum time to start it is within ten years of your last period – the 'window of opportunity' – because our general health risks increase with age. Starting HRT after this should be carefully considered as then some risks such as blood clots, stroke and heart disease can be higher for some women.

The options

There are two primary types of medical hormone treatment: combined HRT, which contains both oestrogen and progesterone, or oestrogen-only. Testosterone (see page 60) can be added into both types. If a woman still has her womb, the combined version is prescribed, as progesterone is needed to balance oestrogen in the womb to reduce the thickening of the womb lining.

HRT comes in lots of different forms: tablets (taken orally), transdermal (meaning through the skin, via gels, spray, cream and patches), pessaries (inserted into the vagina for a more localised dose), creams, rings (inserted into the vagina) and HRT implants, which are usually only available privately. Implants aren't an NHS option because they last for six to twelve months and can't be removed if a woman was diagnosed with a hormone dependent cancer like breast or ovarian cancer.

If you decide on hormone treatment, the regime can take two different forms: the first is sequential, sometimes called cyclical. If you haven't had any surgery and still have your womb, you'll most likely receive your HRT in this way. In perimenopause, women tend to still have periods, which may be irregular. Sequential HRT creates a kind of artificial menstrual cycle, and at the end of each month you will have a withdrawal bleed, a little like you would on some contraceptive pills.

The second way of taking HRT is continuous, which is recommended for women who've had a year without a period and are therefore post-menopausal. It's a 'non-bleed' regime of HRT, so you wouldn't have a period at the end of each month.

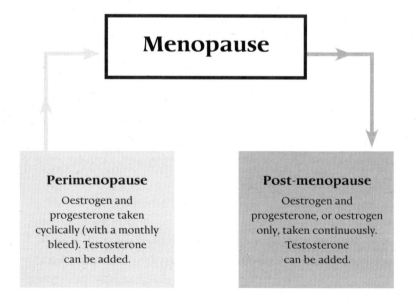

Menopause

Perimenopause

Oestrogen and progesterone taken cyclically (with a monthly bleed). Testosterone can be added.

Post-menopause

Oestrogen and progesterone, or oestrogen only, taken continuously. Testosterone can be added.

HRT REGIMES

Bio-identical versus body-identical HRTs

HRT comes in two forms: bio-identical and body-identical. Bio-identical hormones describe those chemically identical to the ones produced naturally. The bio-identical hormone industry markets itself as the more bespoke and individually tailored, insisting it's more natural than traditional, 'synthetic' HRT. However, it often has to go through some commercial processes (making its claim to be 'natural' slightly questionable) and isn't regulated or used within the NHS, yet women are charged a lot of money for it at some private clinics.

The NHS offers natural, plant-based HRT, often referred to as body-identical. Here's the confusing part: body-identical HRT is bio-identical too, but it's also regulated by the Food and Drug Administration (FDA) in the USA, the European Medicines Agency in Europe, and approved and endorsed by the British Menopause Society and the National Institute of Clinical Excellence (NICE) in the UK.

It's the type of HRT used within the NHS and the type that I advocate because it comes backed by extensive research.

Finding *your* dose

We talk about 'HRT' as if it means one thing but, as you've read so far in this chapter, it can take different forms. Your doctor will assess your needs and advise you on lifestyle changes that can also help to ease your symptoms. A blood test can be done, but isn't always necessary (see page 13). The exception is if you're on progesterone-only contraception, such as the Mirena coil or the implant, because with these methods of contraception most women often don't have periods so a blood test can indicate whether your symptoms are due to perimenopause or one of the other conditions that can mimic it.

It's always best to start HRT cautiously, on a low to moderate dose – the NICE guidelines advise the lowest possible dose to manage symptoms, then more can always be added later if needed. This way there are often fewer side-effects, which can include being bloated, having breast tenderness and feeling nauseous.

Remember, starting HRT is a journey, not a quick fix, and your doctor will work with you to find the right dose to manage your symptoms. Your initial prescription will be reviewed according to your needs, and how your life and medical history changes. It may take a few months to find the correct dose, but often the difference is felt within six to eight weeks.

The NICE guidelines state once you initiate treatment, you should be reviewed at three months then at least annually once you're on a stable dose.

It's not unusual to have an additional appointment at six months – remember, it's not just about what the dose is doing to your body, but your mind, too. And as you age, your body's needs change so it's important to have your hormone treatment reviewed to make adjustments.

Testosterone

Testosterone usually enters the conversation at your second consultation for a few reasons. Firstly, because testosterone's effects are enhanced when you're already on oestrogen; secondly, we want to know how well the oestrogen and progesterone are tackling your symptoms; and thirdly, because at the initial consultation a woman might not have been bothered by symptoms, such as a reduced libido, that can be attributed to declining testosterone because there were other more pressing symptoms at that time.

The mention of specific symptoms – loss of muscle tone, slowing metabolism and weight issues, lack of mental clarity, memory and focus and, yes, a waning libido, would all prompt a discussion around testosterone.

There are exceptions, though, when testosterone might be prescribed from the outset. For example, a patient who, right off the bat, said she couldn't care less if she never had sex again, and it was really affecting her relationship. Ultimately, your HRT prescription will be personalised to suit your needs and your life.

Chicken or egg?

A quarter of women have quite severe and debilitating symptoms that can stop them functioning – they might feel out of control, not recognise themselves and make big lifestyle changes, such as resigning from their job. And the rest of us fall in between.

Perimenopause symptoms can make a lot of women feel demotivated, fatigued, low in mood and lacking in energy. At the same time they may be juggling a career, caring for elderly parents, bringing up children, and dealing with everyday stresses. While they may want to make positive lifestyle adjustments, such as addressing their diet and exercising, they may simply not have the motivation and energy to do so. Starting HRT can give them that motivation and energy to maintain a lifestyle, career and financial independence by giving them back their mental resilience and motivation. Hence my analogy to chicken or egg.

Jennifer's story

When I was 48, I had brain fog, felt constantly overwhelmed, and was finding it hard to cope in my high-pressured role as a senior manager in HR. My memory and focus felt like they'd dissolved and I wondered if I was capable anymore. I was thinking seriously about asking for a demotion – something my 35-year-old self would have been outraged by – or leaving altogether. Feeling like I was at my wit's end, I made an appointment to talk to a menopause doctor about HRT.

Ten weeks later, I went for my review with her feeling like a new woman. I felt lighter, brighter, and sharper – and at work, my fortunes had transformed, so much so I'd actually asked my boss for more work.

Adding those hormones back in boosted my confidence and gave me the physical and mental energy to be the woman I knew I could be. There's the practical side too; my financial independence and wellbeing would have taken a serious hit if I'd acted on my pre-HRT feelings and quit the job I loved. That alone would have affected my quality of life now and into the future. Transitioning onto HRT was the best thing I ever did.

The risks explained

Although taking HRT does come with risks – and it's important to have a full understanding of them – there are some myths, and a whole lot of waffle, so let's do some demystifying.

Twenty years ago, you might have read a headline that screamed, 'HRT doubles your risk of breast cancer' – but note, it was *20 years ago*. At that time, traditional HRT received a lot of bad press because a 2002 study by the Women's Health Initiative (WHI) was stopped after two years due to safety concerns based on its findings. It showed an increased risk of cardiovascular disease and breast cancer in those taking certain types of HRT. The impact was dramatic: the number of women taking HRT dropped drastically.

What was not explained was that the women taking part in the study had a high BMI of 28.5 and an average age of 63, making them ten years post-menopause, outside the critical 'window of opportunity' (see page 57). The results showed that those women who had started HRT close to their menopause had a reduced risk of cardiovascular disease.

The doses used in the trials were also higher than those that are prescribed today. The science behind HRT has moved on a hell of a lot since then, but that doesn't stop myths persisting on the basis of this very old research.

Your lifestyle, the type of HRT, whether you take it orally or through the skin and how long you take it all have an impact on your risk of breast cancer, blood clots and strokes. Giving women HRT in a sequential manner (see page 58) may carry a slightly lower risk of breast cancer than if taken continuously, but obesity is still a higher risk factor.

We want you to be aware of these kinds of nuances because they're key to you feeling as if the information is comprehensive enough for you to make what we know is a big decision. They're what the majority of sensationalised newspaper headlines don't tell you. So, let's take a look at some of the biggest concerns you may have.

Breast cancer

Statistics show that one in eight women will get breast cancer in their lifetime. The biggest risk factors for breast cancer are ageing and being a woman, which we can do

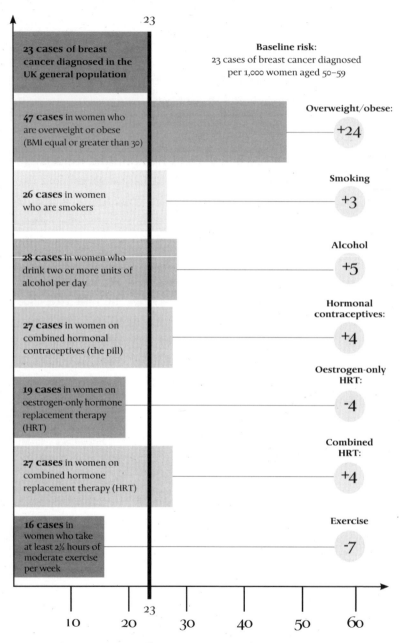

23 cases of breast cancer diagnosed in the UK general population

Baseline risk:
23 cases of breast cancer diagnosed per 1,000 women aged 50–59

47 cases in women who are overweight or obese (BMI equal or greater than 30)

Overweight/obese:
+24

26 cases in women who are smokers

Smoking
+3

28 cases in women who drink two or more units of alcohol per day

Alcohol
+5

27 cases in women on combined hormonal contraceptives (the pill)

Hormonal contraceptives:
+4

19 cases in women on oestrogen-only hormone replacement therapy (HRT)

Oestrogen-only HRT:
-4

27 cases in women on combined hormone replacement therapy (HRT)

Combined HRT:
+4

16 cases in women who take at least 2½ hours of moderate exercise per week

Exercise
-7

10   20   23   30   40   50   60

Breast cancer incidence per 1,000 women aged 50–59

BREAST CANCER RISK FACTORS

nothing about. Around 25 per cent of breast cancers are caused by 'modifiable' lifestyle factors – things we have the power to change, such as our diet and exercise routine. Inherited causes – like those in women who carry the BRCA 1 and 2 genes – account for between 5 and 10 per cent of breast cancers.

So, you can see from the illustraton above where we're going with this – lifestyle factors are important, especially obesity, and it is important to individualise the risks for each woman and put them into perspective for her.

The other big caveat to be aware of is that those statistics lump all HRTs – body-identical, bio-identical, oral, pessaries, sequential, continuous – together. But, as we know, the various forms of HRT are not equal.

Progesterone is the element of HRT that presents a breast cancer risk – not oestrogen. However, 'micronised' progesterone, usually given in capsule form to be taken orally or vaginally, is natural and identical to the progesterone produced by our bodies and it seems not to increase risk. Not all progestogens are equal!

We're still waiting for research to show how all the different types of HRT impact breast cancer risk, but it's very likely studies will show it to be much lower with body-identical HRT. We're not saying women don't get breast cancer because of HRT, but women on HRT have 18 per cent less all-cause cancers than women not on HRT in their lifetime, so it's time to dismiss old headlines and focus on new statistics and studies instead, which paint a very different picture.

Blood clots and strokes

For every 100,000 women *not* on the contraceptive pill, five will have a blood clot. This is what we call a woman's 'baseline risk' of having a blood clot. That risk goes up to 20 in

100,000 for women who are on the contraceptive pill, and up to 60 for pregnant women.

HRT is metabolised in the liver, where clotting factors are produced, and that's why there's an increased risk of blood clots associated with it. It's true taking oral HRT doubles your risk of blood clots, from 10 to 20 cases in 100,000 women, but not as much as during pregnancy when the risk is 60 in 100,000.

However, HRT when applied via the skin (transdermal) and given at the appropriate dose, doesn't increase your risk of blood clots at all. Women with higher risk factors for blood clots – for example being overweight or a smoker, or someone who has perhaps had a provoked blood clot previously (e.g. from trauma) – should be put onto transdermal HRT, rather than an oral one. This is something that would be taken into consideration when medical history is assessed. Yet again, we see how lumping all HRTs together into a single entity isn't actually the best way to give women the information they need to make an educated choice.

Minor risks

For all the pretty heavy risks, we find patients are most concerned with risks and side-effects that could affect them in the here and now – things like bloating, nausea, acne, irregular spotting, palpitations, anxiety and tiredness. These symptoms can occur as your body gets in tune with the additional support, but almost always settle. They are a sign that the body is re-igniting. They aren't major risks, but they matter to women, so it's important to explain what might happen at the outset.

You shouldn't experience 'minor' side-effects like these beyond two to four weeks of taking HRT. While a few women experience weight gain, we would say most don't. Ultimately, if your HRT is in tune with your body, you shouldn't gain fat, but your weight might go up as a result of increasing muscle mass, so when you step on the scales it may say you weigh more, but your clothes will fit you better.

Modifying your risk level

Without wishing to sound too dictatorial, health management and looking after your own health is a joint responsibility; you can't just rely on medication and ignore your lifestyle or diet. HRT confers lots of benefits but, alongside it, you should manage those modifiable risk factors (the ones that cause 25 per cent of breast cancers) that we discussed earlier: not drinking to excess, trying to cut down or stop smoking, eating a balanced diet and doing some exercise. Not doing those things will increase your risk of breast cancer.

HRT alternatives

The NICE guidelines state that HRT should be the first port of call for women with vasomotor symptoms – hot flushes, night sweats, vaginal atrophy (see page 112) or menopausal mood disorder, unless the woman has a reason she can't take HRT, known as a 'contraindication'.

There are some women for whom HRT won't be appropriate; those who have the BRAC gene mutations, which put them at a higher risk of breast cancer, those with oestrogen receptor-positive breast cancer, or women with liver disease.

If you can't, or don't want to, take HRT, there are still plenty of options, supplements and complementary therapies to consider alongside non-hormonal prescription medicines to help you to take charge of your perimenopause (see Chapter 14).

Coming off HRT

During perimenopause, as your ovaries decline in function, your symptoms may become more and more pronounced. In fact, up until your mid- to late-50s your hormones may be fluctuating here, there and everywhere. If you're on HRT, your dose may need to be adjusted accordingly.

But often as your body gets into a rhythm and settles, usually by your mid-50s, you may be able to reduce your HRT prescription. The ovaries of the average woman in her late-50s only produce 1 per cent of the oestrogen they did compared to when she was pre-menopausal so, over time, hormone levels plateau as the body adjusts to the changes.

Women often say, 'But isn't taking HRT just delaying the inevitable?' Translation: 'Won't my perimenopausal symptoms just come flooding back the second I stop taking it?' The answer is no. Carefully managed, that won't happen at all.

If you want to stop taking HRT, discuss it with your doctor and ask for your dose to be tailored down slowly. This will mean that while you might get some symptoms, they'll be nowhere near as florid as those you experienced when you initially started taking HRT. You won't suddenly experience full-blown perimenopausal symptoms.

Staying on HRT

It might surprise you to hear there is no need to come off HRT – *ever!* Some women take it until they're 90. If a woman is feeling good and her health is fine, there's no reason to come off it. We know many women in their 70s who are on HRT. One who stands out in particular was told by her doctor to stop taking replacement hormones. She said, 'I only got married two years ago and I enjoy sex! I don't want to have a dry vagina.' She was delighted to be told by us that she didn't have to if she didn't want to, and that was that.

One of the most commonly held HRT myths is that it can only be taken for a set period of time. Women often say, 'I've heard I can only take it for five years, so I'm going to wait until my symptoms get so bad and save my five years for then.' This perpetuating myth means that many women are missing out and losing their sparkle and worth. There's no need to wait until you feel *really* bad to take HRT because there's no limit to how long you can be on it.

Staying on HRT doesn't mean you'll carry on having periods forever, either. When women start taking HRT as they go through perimenopause, they'll usually start on a sequential treatment plan and have a monthly bleed. Some women actually want to stick with this HRT regime because they like the idea of having a period each month, but many don't. With the average age of menopause being 51 and 90 per cent of women going through it by the time they're 54, at some time between the ages of 50 and 54, we'll switch a woman over to the non-bleed continuous method of HRT. Once this happens, she may get some breakthrough bleeding for a short time, but her periods will ultimately end.

Growing evidence and opinion is that if HRT is started at the right time, the benefits can outweigh the risks for many women in conjunction with a healthy lifestyle, but we would never judge anyone who, armed with the knowledge, chose not to take it. After all, it's one of the most personal choices a woman can make. We want you to feel prepared, not scared, for what's coming your way, and to feel empowered in whatever decision you make.

The bottom line

» Question the myths: so much misinformation persists around HRT, so consider what you think to be true and what you know to be true.

» It's your choice: the decision about whether or not to go on HRT is yours alone.

» Understand the different types of HRT: not all forms are created equal.

» Find your dose: work with your doctor on this, because it will be different to another woman's and may change as you adjust.

» Know the risks: it's important to put the risks into perspective and to understand the context behind the headlines.

» You don't have to come off HRT: but if you want to, discuss the decision with your doctor.

CHAPTER 5

Pro-Ageing

Looking at ageing through a positive lens is more about what you *can* do rather than what you can't.

The visible, outward cosmetic changes that occur during perimenopause can cause women to lose their confidence and their feeling of femininity and sexiness – and it can often seem like it's happened overnight. Factors like skin laxity, age spots, wrinkles, brittle nails and thinning and less shiny hair can all play their part in making us feel like less attractive versions of ourselves. But it doesn't have to be this way. In this chapter, we'll explore the aesthetic shifts that alter our appearance and delve into the solutions.

We might feel silly or shallow for admitting it, but the way our appearance changes during perimenopause has a huge impact on our self-belief and self-esteem. This isn't exactly surprising, so conditioned are we to see getting older as a complete and unmitigated *disaster*.

The narrative that persists around women and ageing is negative – we're portrayed as increasingly shrivelled, dry and grey, until such time as we reach a tipping point beyond which we're no longer sexy. This well-trodden story can make even the steeliest women feel insecure as they age.

The reality is women in midlife are more powerful than they've ever been, but that's not how they're treated. Older female actors are shunted into character roles, whereas men are seen as silver foxes, in their prime. And while the perception of women in middle age is changing, those who seem like they're smashing it (hello, J Lo, Michelle Obama and Jennifer Aniston) seem woefully out of reach to the average woman.

We're also caught in a tug-of-war – we feel a pressure to look good, while simultaneously insisting that we don't care what we look like, for fear of betraying the sisterhood.

We need to be honest and acknowledge the role our outward appearances play in how we feel about ourselves and how society perceives us, and we need to do it without shame or embarrassment. Studies show attractive people are more successful, perceived as more trustworthy and make more money. So don't feel bad about yourself because you want to look good; you can't unpick thousands of years' worth of conditioning. Yes, we're very much a visual society and while we may want to look radiant, we shouldn't allow it to define ourselves. Perimenopause is a time to regain your confidence and become the person you should have been.

Besides, the evidence speaks for itself. Studies show when we think we look good, we feel good, too; and when we feel we look 'bad', it can be terrible for our self-esteem and mental health. Of course, if how you feel about yourself is entirely unconnected to your appearance that's completely liberating, but it's not the lived experience of many women and it would be wrong to deny the huge impact the aesthetic changes brought on by perimenopause have on our emotional wellbeing. Psychologists call this 'appearance contingent self-worth', meaning we value ourselves based on the way we look and, while it'd be a rare person who'd call this ideal, it's what many women call reality.

Despite the mental health implications of feeling bad about how you look, women still feel unable to discuss their concerns with their doctor, for fear of sounding frivolous. After all, feeling down because you're worried about your appearance isn't heart disease or cancer – but it isn't nothing, either.

Many breast cancer survivors say they feel unsupported when it comes to concerns about their post-recovery appearance. They feel guilty for talking about it because, well, they've been cured of their cancer, right? So, to say to their doctor 'my skin feels dry' or 'my hair doesn't feel so lustrous anymore' feels downright silly. But to underestimate women's appearance-based worries is to take a very short-term, shortsighted view of what 'health' really is.

Stop fighting yourself

Ageing is a natural process; we can't deny or defy it, but we can still look and feel our best. The term 'anti-ageing' makes it sound like we're going to take the fight to our naturally ageing bodies. Instead, we want women to feel they *look* good and therefore *feel* good at every life stage – looking the best you can and making proactive life choices is what is meant by pro-ageing. Viewing ageing through a positive lens seems almost radical.

Some might see a contradiction between embracing who you are and making the best of what you have, but we don't. It's all about balance – you can be happy in yourself and simultaneously want to do things that make you feel good. Let's be honest, most women don't actually pine for the body they had when they were 25 – they see the value in their 50-year-old body, which has navigated an extra quarter-century of life's changes – but they want to make the best of the body they have.

The changes outlined

Accept yourself, but don't limit yourself. You have the power to make changes: if there are things you're unhappy about, you'll find the tools to do something about them here.

Your face

Collagen is the main structural protein found in the body's connective tissues. It acts as scaffolding, holding our skin, bones and cartilage in shape.

Our bodies stop producing collagen from around the age of 25. From then onwards, we begin to 'age' in an aesthetic sense, losing collagen at a rate of about 1 per cent per year until the perimenopause, at which time this loss accelerates to about 2–5 per cent per year. Once we've been through the menopause, we'll have lost approximately 30 per cent of our collagen.

The consequences of this shift are well documented: the lack of collagen causes the face to sag and lose its structure and frame. Alongside that, perimenopause causes the face to lose fat – and therefore volume – and the bones to lose density.

Oestrogen is responsible for the production of elastin, another protein that allows our skin to return to its former shape after stretching or contracting. Once oestrogen starts to decline, so too do our levels of elastin, and our skin loses the plumpness it once had.

In short, these factors combine to cause our faces to slide into an upside down 'V' shape as they age. You might feel like your cheeks are less full, your jawline less defined, that jowls start to develop. The skin itself also gets thinner, drier and begins to display more lines and wrinkles. Many women see the impact of these hormonal changes in their lips, which become thinner and less full, giving that pursed lip effect.

The under-eye area is the other part of the face where changes are pronounced. We can develop 'crows feet' and show obvious signs of hormone-induced sleep issues. Facial skin can also fall victim to pigmentation – women report an increase in freckles, lentigos (age spots) due to sun damage and hyperpigmentation, known as melasma, where patches of skin become darker in colour than the skin around them due to hormonal imbalance.

The eyes may become drier, more sensitive to light and itchy because, just like the rest of our bodies, we've lost some of that natural lubrication layer on the surface. Also have you noticed your eyesight has changed? Are you now wearing reading glasses? Some of this is due to the change in eye shape that occurs with natural ageing, but also to declining oestrogen levels affecting the muscles and ligaments around the eye.

As if this wasn't enough, some women find acne becomes a problem during perimenopause. This is caused by the 'androgenic', or masculine, effects of testosterone (which can become more dominant for some woman as their oestrogen levels dip) and the increased production of sebum.

Studies have shown that women in their 40s get more acne nowadays than they might have done 30 years ago because they're living more stressful lives. The relative prominence of testosterone can also cause increased facial hair. If you've noticed the odd hair or cluster of hairs sprouting on your chin, this is why. It's not that we suddenly have more testosterone; it's because we have less of the female hormones oestrogen and progesterone, so testosterone can be more powerful in its effects than it was pre-menopause. For more information on acne, its causes and what you can do about it turn to page 211.

Your body

Changes in collagen and elastin mean the skin on your body will undergo the same changes as your facial skin. Declining testosterone also prompts muscle loss (called sarcopenia), meaning the skin that was once stretched taut around those muscles loosens. This is usually most obvious in areas like the neck and upper arms. Hormonal decline can also have a visible impact on specific areas of the body:

Your breasts: a drop in progesterone makes the breast tissue less ductile and more fatty, which causes the breasts to become heavier and start to sag. Again, the lack of collagen and elastin makes the skin less elastic and taut.

Your waist: declining hormones and increased insulin resistance can cause women's waistlines to become less defined during perimenopause. This is sometimes referred to as 'the middle age spread'. For more information on the causes and what you can do about it, see page 162.

Your vagina: lower levels of collagen and elastin affect all parts of our bodies, including the vulva and vagina. Women report their vulvas begin to look 'crepey', drier and sometimes pigmented. There is less pubic hair and what is there will start to grey.

Your hands: many women notice the signs of ageing in their hands, sometimes before they see them in their face. Your nails might become brittle and flakey, while the skin on your hands tends to dry. You might notice age spots and your hands looking more veiny due to thinning skin.

Your hair

Women get particularly upset over what hormonal decline does to their crowning glory. Somehow, our hair is intimately connected to how attractive we feel. Blame Pantene, blame L'Oreal, but many of us just don't feel 'worth it' when our hair goes from lustrous to limp.

The decline in oestrogen causes women to shed their hair more frequently, usually evenly all over their scalp, rather than in patches (as can happen with alopecia sufferers). Hair becomes generally dry and brittle and doesn't grow to its former lengths, seeming to break off in ways it might not have before.

There are other factors that contribute to hair changing: as part of the normal ageing process, our hair follicles flatten, our hair shafts thin, and melanin changes cause both men and women's hair to grey. Before you explore aesthetic solutions to hair issues, check in with your doctor because these symptoms can also be caused by other issues, including hypothyroidism (an underactive thyroid), low iron levels or stress. Bear in mind that any remedy is going to take time to work – it takes approximately nine months to see the positive effects of hair growing back. For a deeper dive into hair thinning, see page 212.

What you can do

Looking at ageing through a positive lens is all about thinking what you *can* do rather than what you can't – and some of those things are incredibly simple. As always, the spectrum of options ranges from medication to lifestyle changes to more invasive treatments. Some will feel like a sensible next step, while other suggestions might seem downright scary. Our advice? Read on with an open mind and your self-esteem will reap the rewards.

Here are a few simple lifestyle changes for starters:

» Eating a healthy, balanced diet with good fats, plenty of vegetables and fruit, and less refined sugars and processed food will show in your face.
» Exercise improves circulation and muscle tone, helping to bring that glow and luminosity back. It also helps you to destress, so reduces that permanent frown on your face.
» Stay hydrated. So many of us forget to drink enough water during the day and have lots of dehydrating drinks, such as coffee or tea.
» Simply smiling will give you a more youthful appearance.
» Use drops when your eyes are feeling tired.
» If you're feeling puffy in the face, then it's time to cut back on alcohol.
» Try to get a good night's sleep (see Chapter 8).
» If you smoke, STOP!

Switch up your skincare regime

If you've been using the same moisturiser since your 20s, now is the time to take a long, hard look at your bathroom cabinet. The skin we have now is not the skin we had then, and you need products to match. You don't have to spend a lot – there are great skincare brands to suit all budgets.

Retinol: this is now in many skincare brands of all price ranges. A member of the vitamin A family, retinol was originally taken orally as a treatment for acne, and has only recently been marketed as an ingredient in serums and creams that can help with older skin. It works by increasing cell turnover, which improves the appearance of fine lines and wrinkles. Retinol makes the skin photosensitive, so don't use it in the daytime. Instead, apply it at night before you go to sleep. At first, use it every other night and then build up, because it can be harsh on the skin, making it flaky, dry and red initially.

Vitamin C: this is another key component of any perimenopausal woman's skincare regime because it helps pep up the skin and inject brightness. Choose a product (usually in the form of a serum) with 10–15 per cent vitamin C (ascorbic acid) on the label, wear it during the day, and you'll soon find you have some of your old glow back. To increase your dietary intake of vitamin C, see page 166.

Sunscreen: this is essential to protect the skin from free radicals (a term that describes unstable atoms that can damage skin cells). UV radiation causes the production of free radicals, so make sure your sunscreen protects against UBV rays, which cause sunburn, and UVA, which penetrate more deeply and are behind much premature skin ageing. Adequate sun protection also works wonders when it comes to preventing pigmentation of the facial skin. We suggest wearing it all year round – just because the sky isn't blue doesn't mean your skin won't be damaged by UV rays.

Moisturising: like facial skin, the skin on our bodies, including our vulvas, can become dry and itchy, so it's important to make body moisturising a concrete part of your post-shower or pre-bedtime routine. You don't have to opt for an expensive brand – look out for ingredients like glycerine, ceramides and humectants. Using a simple coconut oil and even baby oil applied onto damp skin stepping out of the shower works. French pharmacy brands are brilliant reasonably priced options. La Roche Posay, Avene and Vichy all get the thumbs up from us and many dermatologists we know.

Smoking and drinking alcohol

Like the sun's UV rays, smoking creates free radicals that break the bonds in the skin, accelerating the ageing process long before 'normal' decline. It creates wrinkles, including lines around the mouth, and dries the skin. We're not exaggerating when we say that quitting smoking is one of the most positive pro-ageing steps you can take. Some surgeons actively ask their patients to stop smoking before an operation to help speed up the skin's healing process.

Alcohol causes puffiness, bloating and broken capillaries, so drink in moderation – less than 14 units per week, which equates to seven single measures of gin and tonic.

Give yourself a refresh and reboot

In the past, the rules of ageing seemed to dictate that every woman over 45 must chop her hair into a bob and take her miniskirts to the charity shop.

We say: no!

There are *zero* rules at this age and you don't have to abide by any conventions, but if you've lost touch with your hair, wardrobe and make-up bag, there's plenty you can do to make yourself look and feel better.

Take a look at your clothes. Are you still wearing things you bought 20 years ago? Are you really – honestly – wearing the right dress size? Many women find if they go up a size, their clothes fit dramatically better, and they feel much better as a result.

One thing we would definitely recommend is to get your boobs measured and buy the best bras you can afford. Wearing a good supportive bra that is the right size can make all the difference and will improve your posture, especially if perimenopause has caused your body shape to change. This is what we mean by embracing yourself and being proactive – accept the body you have, rather than yearning for the one you once had, then make it look its best.

Don't underestimate the power of having the right products and knowing what to do with them.

Here are some pointers that can work wonders for boosting confidence:

» Revisit your haircut and colour: pay for the best you can afford. As TV presenter Cat Deeley said, 'I could have the latest shoes or the It bag of the season, but my hair is what I wear all the time.'
» Invest in a good primer to help prep your skin and even out skin tone.
» Use an under-eye highlighter or concealer because the under-eye skin gets thinner and isn't helped by a lack of sleep.
» Use over-the-counter eye drops to moisturise your eyes, and if you spend a lot of time in front of a screen, set yourself a reminder to blink and look away to relax those eye muscles.
» Don't ignore your eyebrows: they frame your face. Invest in a good eyebrow pencil or powder, or for the more permanent look, get them tinted or micro-bladed.

» Think weightless, breathable cream formulas rather than matt/powdered make-up. They add a luminosity and radiance that perimenopausal skin can often lack.

» Sometimes less is more when it comes to midlife make-up. Use a light foundation or tinted moisturiser, mascara and lip tint or plumper.

Try a 'tweakment'

We've all seen tabloid pictures of so-called cosmetic surgery 'disasters' – trout pouts, expressionless faces and stretched skin. The perception these images create of any cosmetic enhancements being a short route to looking ridiculous, as well as their cost, has caused some women to dismiss certain categories of beauty treatment altogether.

That said, cosmetic surgery is a broad brush and at the less invasive end of the scale are a number of treatments women you most likely know are using on the quiet. They'll be your colleagues and friends who look great, but not scary. The ones who seem to have an inner luminosity. They don't look abnormal, or like they've 'had work done', they just look amazing, and you find yourself wondering, 'What's her secret?' Let us clue you in: it might be injectables, lasers, filler, Botox or a combination of them all.

A lot of people feel iffy about these types of treatment, but they are slowly losing their stigma, largely thanks to the women who do have them being more open about it. It's no longer seen as 'anti-feminist' or 'shallow' to want to feel better about yourself. Even Caitlin Moran, one of feminism's leading lights, recently outed herself as a Botox convert. Some women are hesitant about putting something they perceive as 'foreign' into their body, but most injectables are made of hyaluronic acid, a natural substance that already exists in our skin. Botox is also used medically for conditions like hyperhidrosis (excess sweating), migraine and having an overactive bladder, so it's not just for cosmetic use. If you're nervous about trying it, but want to give it a go, you can start at a low dose and be reassured that it isn't permanent – it wears off after 3–4 months.

These types of treatments – or 'tweakments' – can create a calmer and less stony look. They make the face appear more relaxed and reinvigorate the skin. During perimenopause, women often feel like they're in a tug-of-war between their face and their body – if they lose weight, will their face become more gaunt? Or do they keep weight on to make their face look fuller? But it doesn't have to be a trade-off – there's a way to achieve balance. In the interests of full disclosure, we've both dabbled with Botox, filler, fractional radio frequency, micro-needling and Profhilo – a type of injectable moisturiser sometimes dubbed the 'liquid facelift'.

Within this category of slightly more intensive treatments, we'd include laser hair removal. Many women find waxing, shaving, depilatory creams and tweezing suffice for their hair removal needs (and no, the irony of developing facial hair while losing the hair on our heads is not lost on us), but lasers can provide a longer-lasting solution. There's no permanent way of removing hair and the expense of laser treatment can be off-putting, but if excess hair is a primary issue for you and you can afford it, it's worth considering. Many clinics offer a payment plan.

Finally, it's worth mentioning that vaginal laser treatments are an extremely effective way to help with vaginal laxity, urinary leakage, vaginal dryness and recurrent UTIs. It's a painless treatment that works by stimulating new collagen and increasing blood flow.

Whatever you choose – if anything at all – it's all about making the right choice for you. Maybe a good skincare regime, eating a healthy diet and exercising (with all its endorphin-releasing, circulation-boosting, muscle-building power) is enough to make you feel good – to age positively.

If you're considering exploring these treatments, always go to a qualified practitioner, doctor or nurse and don't opt for the cheapest.

The bottom line

» You're not shallow or vain: caring about your appearance is completely natural.

» Stop fighting yourself: ageing is a natural process – we can't deny or defy it, but we can do it well and still look and feel our best.

» Be aware of the changes: you'll likely see the signs of ageing in your face, body, vagina and hair.

» Revamp: it's time to overhaul your wardrobe and make sure you're wearing the right bra.

» There's lots you can do: a whole spectrum of options awaits – from revamping your make-up bag to trying a 'tweakment'.

CHAPTER 6

Mind Matters

Discovering any mental health struggles you've been having are the result of perimenopausal hormone shifts can feel surprisingly empowering.

Women often find their mental health takes a hit during perimenopause and the psychological impact this life stage can have is often underestimated. Menopausal women are often referred to as moody, unstable and irrational and numerous studies have looked at mood disturbances during the menopause transition. Hormonal changes and decline are often to blame and even if you haven't experienced anxiety in the past, you may find you feel anxious, panicky, low and lacklustre. While menopausal mood disorder (MMD) is not a formal diagnosis on its own, it's real. Unfortunately, few women know about it, so they struggle on. Those that do go to their doctor (a giant leap in itself) may walk away with a prescription for antidepressants. When you don't know why these changes are occurring, it's easy to feel like you're losing yourself, so in this chapter we'll look at why these shifts in mood happen and give you the tools to cope.

When we talk about perimenopause as all hot flushes and night sweats, we're doing ourselves a disservice, because the hormonal decline women experience during perimenopause can have profound consequences for our mental health, too.

The stark reality is that it's no coincidence the average age of menopause is 51 and rates of suicide in women are highest amongst women aged 45–54; the time when there is a reduction in the level of ovarian hormones during the menopause transition. It's not surprising that divorce rates are highest for women aged 40–45. Of course, there are lots of reasons women might experience mental health or relationship issues – after all these things can happen at any age, but we might be ignoring perimenopausal contributions to these figures.

Let's be clear: the hormonal changes happening to our physical bodies can have long-lasting, far-reaching and life-changing consequences for our mental wellbeing, and therefore every aspect of our lives.

While discussion of perimenopause tends to focus on the physical signs, the mental and emotional symptoms can creep in silently. In fact, in the early stage of perimenopause, when periods are normal and you might not know anything is even happening, the psychological symptoms can be at their most pronounced.

Midlife is a stage when women are juggling many balls and at the same time may be feeling sad and dissatisfied. It's also a reflective period. They might think: 'What have I achieved?' or, 'Where am I going?' and experience a sense of loss and invisibility.

A woman may notice she has had two periods in one month and connect the dots to the perimenopause, but when it comes to feelings of flatness, anxiety and forgetfulness she may not assume the same.

When a woman forgets why she went upstairs or doesn't remember where she put her car keys, she's more likely to think she's getting dementia before she attributes those things to the perimenopause. Nonetheless, those seemingly small things might begin to escalate, affecting her self-esteem and undermining her confidence at work, and as a partner, friend and parent.

Although studies have also linked perimenopause to anxiety, depression and a worsening of existing depressive symptoms, changes in mood during perimenopause can be distinctive from other mental health issues, so let's examine what happens to our emotional wellbeing during this especially sensitive time.

Menopausal mood disorder (MMD)

When considering what happens to our hormones during perimenopause, it's useful to think of the macro- and micro-pictures simultaneously. The perimenopause, the process leading up to menopause, can take many years and describes a time when our hormones are broadly decreasing (that's the macro bit). But while the overall trend is one of decline, our hormones fluctuate during this time, meaning on some days they might be at pre-menopausal levels. These more granular, micro-shifts might sound small, but they are noteworthy.

Oestrogen is responsible for maintaining the brain's levels of our 'happy hormones' – serotonin, noradrenaline and dopamine. It behaves like our body's own internal antidepressant, working to prevent the depletion and degradation of those hormones. So far, so straight forward, right? On days when you feel fabulous, your oestrogen levels – and therefore your happy chemicals – will be relatively normal. But on other days, you'll feel low and lacking in purpose, and that's when oestrogen and your happy chemicals will have taken a dip.

You might not necessarily feel depressed – just a bit flat, like you've lost your zest for life and everything feels like hard work; often women tell me it's like walking uphill or wading through treacle. Perimenopausal women often say they can continue working and socialising, but after a 'fun' activity, like going for a coffee with friends, they want to have a lie down.

This might progress to multiple days when all you want to do is lie on the sofa and watch Netflix, but it's when these days become more regular than your 'up' days that meno-pausal mood disorder (MMD) becomes a concern.

Women with MMD find their anxiety reaches a point where it feels debilitating and out of control, but they don't tend to feel sad consistently. Simple things you'd do without thinking twice about before – like deciding what to cook for dinner or driving – can feel overwhelming.

Many women say, 'I've been driving for 25 years, but I don't want to go on the motorway anymore.' They've lost their confidence and decisiveness. Work tasks might once have taken 20 minutes now take an hour, because they're now double- or triple-checking their every move.

Physical symptoms can cause emotional distress and exac-erbate MMD, too – disrupted sleep might be behind lower concentration levels, for example, and hot flushes can induce feelings of shame. In women who've never experienced anxi-ety before, this can be a scary time, and women with obsessive compulsive disorder (OCD), or a tendency towards OCD-type behaviours, usually find these become more pronounced.

What you can do

Making lifestyle changes, such as having a prescriptive approach to exercise, with two 15-minute sessions a day morning and evening, has shown to improve mild to moderate mood disorders. Also eating healthily for your mood and looking after your gut health (see Chapter 12) – the gut produces 70 per cent of our happy hormone serotonin, so eating the right foods and looking after our gut microbiome will work wonders for our mental health. If mood changes are hormonal, ideally you won't be put on antidepressants but if you are, for any reason, it doesn't mean you have failed.

Jane's story

I'm a 46-year-old garden designer and run my own award-winning landscaping business. From the outside, I appeared successful but, a few years ago, I started to doubt myself. I struggled to assess my own value and price my work, and each job was taking progressively longer. I wasn't perpetually sad, but on an increasing number of days I found myself feeling a bit low. My children, who were 21 and 19, complained I failed to remember things they told me, and the family were forever dismissing my anger as hypersensitivity, or 'crying wolf'. I had been to see my doctor, who offered me antidepressants, but I knew I wasn't depressed, I'd been depressed in the past and this wasn't the same, and anyway, what was it that I should be depressed about? I was trying to exercise regularly, but just didn't have the motivation and drive, and was snacking throughout the day for comfort and to boost energy. My weight creeping up was making me more anxious.

I now understand that this was due to hormonal changes. I wasn't depressed; this was menopausal mood disorder, which happens because of the drop in oestrogen having a knock-on effect and my brain having less of the happy chemicals it was used to. I wasn't keen to start HRT, but had to do something. When I was younger I'd had an eating disorder and I didn't want this situation to get out of control. Right now I wasn't in a mentally strong place nor had I the energy to make the changes to my diet and lifestyle. I was stuck in a rut.

I soon started to feel better, and started going running again, which had always in the past been my go-to mood elevator. I've decided to stay on a low dose of HRT to help level out my hormones, but am also paying more attention to my diet and having some downtime for me. I'm more decisive and valuing myself when I price my jobs. My husband has also commented that I no longer repeatedly keep checking the back door to see if I've locked it and my children have noticed I'm calmer and more receptive.

Higher risk factors

There are some factors that are proven to exacerbate the mood changes brought on by declining oestrogen. If you've experienced one or more of the below, you'll be more susceptible to and at higher risk of mood disturbances during the menopause transition:

» A past history of depression and/or anxiety
» Postnatal depression
» PMS/PMT/PMDD
» Life trauma, such as the loss of a partner or child, or experience of abuse

Previous experience of mental health issues is perhaps the biggest risk factor for experiencing MMD. If you've had mental health issues before, they're likely to rear their head again during this time, which is why it's so important to be perimenopause-aware. Keep your symptoms checklist in mind (see page 23), and if you're starting to experience some of the psychological ones, make an appointment with your doctor. Don't forget you can self-refer for talking therapies (see page 95).

Often, though, women who've had mental health problems are the first to realise how they felt during a past depressive episode is very different to how they feel now. They'll say, 'I don't feel right, but this doesn't feel like the depression I had in my late twenties.' The difference is most likely due to the impact of reduced oestrogen. When people experience depression early on in life, it's often what's called a 'reactive' depression – a depressive episode directly related to a life event. But MMD isn't triggered by a traumatic incident. Instead, it's what we might call a chemical event, caused by hormonal changes. That's why it can feel different to other mental health issues you may have confronted in the past.

Distinguishing MMD from other mental health conditions

Studies show mental health issues of almost all kinds increase during perimenopause, such as:

» Depression
» Anxiety disorders (which include generalised anxiety disorder, post-traumatic stress disorder and panic disorder)
» Phobias

» Disordered eating (including anorexia, bulimia and binge-eating disorder)
» Addiction, such as alcohol – often used as a crutch by women during this time to alleviate anxiety and sleep problems
» Obsessive compulsive disorder (OCD)

It is important to understand that we all have 'mental health', and as a society we're becoming more aware that we must take as much care of it as we do our physical health.

You might already have inkling as to what extent your perimenopausal hormone changes are responsible for how you feel. MMD is most commonly misdiagnosed as depression but, as we know, with MMD, your mood will fluctuate. At times, you might not want to dress up and go dancing, but that despondency won't feel permanent. Instead, sufferers of depression experience consistently low mood for two weeks, early morning waking, over or under-eating, slowing down of thought and movement and anhedonia – the medical term for a complete loss of interest in things that you usually would enjoy.

If you're concerned you might be depressed, your doctor may ask you to fill out a questionnaire (see page 287). Try doing it in advance and write down your scores to discuss with your doctor.

It's possible that your mental health symptoms are not MMD and you could have generalised anxiety disorder or depression. This, however, is more likely if you have a past history of mental health problems or a stressful life event, such as redundancy or bereavement, knocks you off course during perimenopause.

Of course, it's possible to be diagnosed with *both* MMD and another mental health condition simultaneously. Panic disorder is common among perimenopausal women, who might get panic attacks when in crowds, or when faced with doing something they've always been accustomed to doing, such as driving on a motorway.

Sometimes, there might be a web of conflicting causes and effects – for example, a woman whose hormones cause her to underperform at work and lose her job, who then experiences a bout of reactive depression as a result. It is important to untangle what is due to 'life' and what is due to hormones.

Life stresses

In our experience, particularly in early perimenopause, when physical symptoms like hot flushes and night sweats haven't arrived yet, women tend to attribute their mental health concerns to, for example, their stressful job, difficult relationship, ill parents or teenage children. These things are challenging, but you might ordinarily be able to cope with them were it not for your swirling perimenopausal hormones. For example, if you're waking up in the morning thinking, 'What's the point of getting out of bed?', it's not because your children have gone to university (even though you might have decided that's the cause), it's because this life event has happened while your hormones aren't as stable as they once were. You would feel far more resilient and able to cope with everyday stresses if you weren't enduring the hormonal changes caused by the perimenopause at the same time.

Treatments and solutions

Discovering any mental health struggles you've been having are the result of perimenopausal hormone shifts can feel surprisingly empowering and getting your mind back on track can mark a new beginning.

When it comes to tackling the range of mental health issues occurring during perimenopause, there's no silver bullet. There is, however, a range of options, depending on whether you're dealing with MMD, another condition, or a combination of the two. The type of treatment will also depend on the severity of your symptoms. Diet, exercise and stress management are all pivotal on their own and in parallel with any medical intervention.

Diet

When you're feeling low, you may tend to reach for carbo-hydrates and other high-sugar foods, so be aware of your personal triggers. Eat nutrient-dense food regularly through-out the day to maintain your food intake and energy balance. Not eating will depress your mood and further suppress the release of those happy hormones. Women sometimes treat alcohol as a crutch to help calm their anxiety or bring on sleep, but while it might feel good in the short-term, alcohol feeds into the anxiety and depression cycle and exacerbates symptoms. Cut back on alcohol (and caffeine, for the same reason). For more information on eating to beat meno-pausal symptoms, see Chapter 11.

Exercise

You might hate the thought of exercise, but reframing it as 'movement' can help. It doesn't have to be running in the rain or slogging out a HIIT workout (although if you like those things, great – perhaps it's putting on some Beyoncé and dancing around your kitchen. Whatever it is, pitch it at the right level: you want to be able to talk when you're doing it, but not sing. This type of 'moderate intensity' exer-cise will give you a release of endorphins without leaving you feeling totally exhausted. Better still, research shows that the buoyant chemical effect of ten minutes of physical activity will stay with you for hours afterwards. For more information on exercise, see Chapter 13.

Therapy

There are many different types of therapy to help women navigate both MMD and other mental health issues. Doing some introspective work during the transitional stage of perimenopause can be transformative.

Women report simply having some time to themselves works wonders, and they also say it helps to unpick any long-standing thought patterns that might be preventing them from moving forwards. For those at higher risk of mental health issues because they've endured a traumatic event, therapy at this point (whether they've tried it before, but especially if they haven't) can really help.

Below is a list of some of the different types of therapies available, which you can ask your doctor for on the NHS or directly access privately. Waiting times for NHS therapy might be a little longer than you'd like. You can access counselling via the website mentioned on page 299.

Counselling/therapy: talking to a counsellor/therapist in confidence about a variety of issues can help patients to understand why they are feeling a particular way and find ways to deal with those issues. There are many different types of counselling/therapy. One commonly used for depression and anxiety is cognitive behavioural therapy (CBT). A therapist works with you to look at your thoughts and behaviours and find ways to address and break any negative patterns (see diagram below).

Emotional freedom techniques (EFT): EFT, which is often described as 'tapping therapy', uses practices from

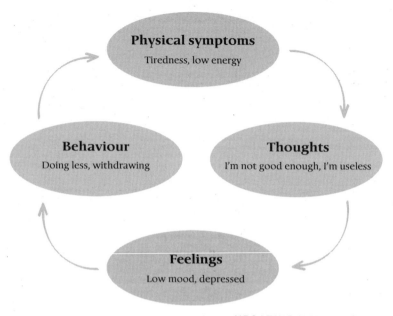

NEGATIVE MENTAL CYCLE

alternative medicine, like acupuncture, to help patients deal with their fears by applying touch to different parts of the body. Proponents believe that EFT can create balance and treat emotional pain.

Group therapy: if you're open to the idea, group therapy can make people feel less alone in their struggles.

Mindfulness: 'mindfulness' has become one of those eye-roll-inducing words, because it has been overused to the point where it has lost its meaning. It can, however, help to calm and reduce stress when you are on the treadmill of life. It is especially helpful for women in peri-menopause who are often rushing around, multi-tasking and functioning on autopilot. Mindfulness techniques, whether practised through formal meditation techniques, or informally, such as eating more mindfully or staying in the moment as you go about your daily tasks, help you to slow down, focus and be aware of and handle all your feelings, including the negative ones.

> ### How to find a therapist
>
> To find an accredited local therapist, go to the British Association for Counselling and Psychotherapy (BACP) website (see page 299) and search by entering your postcode. The British Menopause Society can be a useful place to find a therapist who deals more specifically with issues around menopause.

Community

Social media gets a bad rep when it comes to the impact it has on our mental health, but the ease with which it enables us to find people going through similar experiences is one of its big positives. Lots of Facebook groups and Instagram accounts have really opened up the conversation around mental health. Talking to a community of like-minded women (many of whom share much more candidly than you might expect) can help you to feel less isolated.

Medication

A natural alternative to HRT is St John's Wort, an over-the-counter herbal remedy. Research suggests it can help improve mild to moderate mental health issues by increasing the production of those happy chemicals, namely serotonin and noradrenaline. It can, however, interact with and hamper the effectiveness of the contraceptive pill and anti-epileptic medication. Speak to your doctor before you begin taking it if you have any concerns.

Starting on a low dose of HRT may help prevent the fluctuation of hormone levels that causes MMD, even for those women who were sensitive to the 'pill'. This is because the oestrogen in HRT is at a much lower dose and the same as 90 per cent of the oestrogen naturally produced by the body, whereas the pill contains a synthetic version. For those women who are sensitive to progesterone, the first HRT prescribed may need to be changed to find the one that suits them.

Choosing to take HRT doesn't mean you have 'given in' – there are lots of benefits of starting low and building up gradually as more perimenopausal symptoms come into play. Although declining oestrogen levels wreak the most havoc, progesterone has a role in the neurochemistry of our brain, especially on the receptors responsible for calmness and sleep. If a lack of sexual desire is playing into your MMD symptoms, you might also want to include libido and energy-boosting testosterone (see page 60) in your HRT prescription. As this can be difficult to get hold of from your regular NHS GP, if necessary ask for a referral to a local menopause clinic or seek out another doctor in your practice who is more aware.

Other types of medication can be taken in conjunction with HRT – or on their own – to alleviate specific issues. Beta-blockers slow the heart rate and can be taken as and when they're needed if panic attacks or anxiety are sometimes a problem for you.

Another treatment option is a prescription for antidepressant medication. Selective serotonin reuptake inhibitors (SSRIs) are the most common type of antidepressant and they act by preventing the brain from breaking down our key stabilising happy hormone, serotonin, which stops our levels from dropping. The NICE guidelines say that antidepressants shouldn't be used to treat MMD in the first instance. Consider HRT if not contraindicated, but don't forget diet, exercise and therapy all play their role. That said, antidepressants shouldn't be ruled out, particularly if a significant life event happens in parallel to perimenopause.

Jabeen's story

At 46, I was in a loving relationship of eight years with my partner. I'd always had PMT so she was used to my monthly outbursts, but she'd noticed I seemed angrier at times. At work, I was getting irritated by the smallest of things and finding it difficult to motivate myself, but then some days I was back to being my usual self. I was finding more and more I didn't want to go out and felt tired all the time. I preferred having 'duvet days' watching Netflix rather than socialising. My partner finally confronted me and said I was no fun anymore, and that was the tipping point.

I went to see my doctor and she asked me a series of questions, including if my periods had changed. I told her they had and that life just seemed hard work, like having constant PMT. I knew what depression was like – I'd gone through a period of it and this didn't feel the same. She did some blood tests and suggested I start HRT to help balance my hormones. I sort of said yes for my girlfriend's sake. At my review, I was surprised how much better I felt, I think I must have been miserable for a few years and my poor girlfriend had been putting up with it. It's amazing the difference levelling and balancing hormones can make. I don't think I would have believed anyone if I hadn't felt the difference myself.

Katherine's story

I was prompted by my husband to seek help when I was 49 because he believed my moods were taking a toll on our relationship. He was convinced my mood change was down to my hormones. I, however, didn't think it was. My periods were still regular, but I was fed up and consistently down in the dumps. The sexual side of our relationship had vanished – if I'm honest, I just didn't want to be touched by him. I didn't think it was anything to do with my hormones; I thought I was just fed up with him and our relationship, but for his sake and for clarity I decided to get my hormones checked. I was fit and well, exercised regularly and had recently turned vegetarian so I was doing all the right things, but before I threw away 25 years of marriage I thought it was important to eliminate perimenopause as a cause. I thought I'd try 2–3 months of HRT to see if that changed anything.

When nothing changed, I realised I'd been right – my hormonal shift hadn't been playing a major role in my low mood. Nonetheless, balancing my hormones provided me with that clarity to make some life decisions. I booked and started therapy sessions and decided to move out of the family home to give myself some space to work out what I needed and wanted for the next stage of my life. We are also going for couples counselling and currently I'm not sure where this will lead, but I'm thinking for myself for once.

Making big decisions

Women have a habit of making some pretty big decisions during perimenopause (if in doubt, just re-read those divorce rates). For many women it is the catalyst needed to put an end to a relationship that is simply no longer working for them. Whether it's tiny tweaks or major life shifts, now is as good a time as any to re-evaluate your relationships and where they're going. Our advice, though, is to deal with one thing at a time. You're not likely to solve years of grievances overnight and it's always wise to make sure your hormones are as level as possible – and that balance is sustained – before embarking on massive life changes.

If you're mulling over a life-changing decision, stop for a second and don't do anything drastic. In the same way perimenopausal hormone patterns can make our mental health fluctuate, they can also make how we feel about certain issues change from one day or week to the next. Often we make spontaneous decisions based on how we're feeling on a particular day, but on another day your hormones might make you feel differently. Had you acted on either day, you might later have come to regret it.

The same advice goes to women who are depressed – take steps to recalibrate your mood before you act. Then, once you feel more balanced, give it at least three months before you make your move. If you still feel the same way, then it's the right decision.

Managing relationships with others

It can be very hard to open up about what you're experiencing through perimenopause, especially if you don't completely understand it yourself. Perimenopause is hard to pin down at the best of times: it's confusing, ever-shifting, quite often invisible. So, while you may be feeling a seismic shift inside, your family and friends are more than likely unsuspecting and oblivious to the tumult you might be dealing with.

Hormone turbulence can make you feel pretty disconnected from the world. Both of us, in our own ways, found the early stages of perimenopause – before we'd really sussed what was happening – incredibly isolating. It's common for women to distance themselves from their friends and family, sometimes because they don't think others will understand what they're going through, but often because it's not easy to put into words what they're experiencing.

Offloading with female friends

Pick friends who you're close to and who you feel will 'get' it. Don't worry if some meet you with blank stares or if others just don't want to know. Some women might not want to talk about the transition to menopause; they feel like it's admitting defeat or it makes them feel old or past it. Others might be in denial or simply not want to accept that it's happening – even if it's screamingly obvious to you and everyone else. And let's not forget, some women glide through without any issues or symptoms at all, which might impact their ability to empathise. Everyone travels down this path at their own perimenopause pace; we have to be accepting of that.

You may find it's a time when you take stock of your friendships. One woman told us she decided to gently let go of those in her life who she felt didn't give back. It was, she recounts, 'not without guilt at first, but ultimately I felt liberated and I now have zero regrets'. Indeed, the dawnings of perimenopause are far-reaching. Many women feel stronger, braver, more comfortable in their own skin and a lot less inclined to put up with other people's shit. Is it wisdom, because you've been round the block a few times and you're now pretty adept at seeing people for what they really are? Is it the feel-good effects of oestrogen? Who knows, it's probably a combination, but essentially, you realise your 'lady forgiveness' (as brilliantly coined by Caitlin Moran) reserves are in short supply. So, any repeat offenders – the ones who are religiously late, self-centred or never put their hand in their pocket – are likely to get short shrift!

Talking to kids

The fact that menopause is now part of PSHE education in secondary schools will hopefully mean teenagers soon have a better understanding or will at least have heard the term 'perimenopause'. In the meantime, don't try to hide your symptoms; it's an extra layer of stress you simply do not need.

Teenagers are very likely to be going through their own hormonal upheaval, which adds an extra layer of complication, but also a chance to bond – stick with me here. Be open and honest with them. Break it down into small chunks; they don't need to know everything all at once. And drip-feed information where you can. Look out for what are known as teachable moments – in the car is a good one. Reassure your kids it's totally natural and pitch perimenopause like we do, as a kind of reverse puberty. Draw some parallels with what they're going through. It's a pretty wild ride for both of you: acne, mood swings and low self-esteem might suddenly be mutual hot topics for discussions and tips. Encouraging teens to take stock of their health – just like you're doing – makes it into a shared venture and can be a good way to connect. Make it factual rather than a big heart to heart. And choose a time when you're feeling calm, rather than socking it to them in the middle of an argument. If you have a partner, you might even get them to broach the subject with them first.

If, like many women, you have had your children in later life, they might be young during the perimenopausal years. Don't be afraid to reach out and ask for help if you need it and, as necessary, let your children know how you are feeling. Use age-appropriate language, such as 'Mummy is having a bad day today' or 'Mummy just needs some quiet time'.

Sarah's story

I felt weighed down for the longest time.

Perimenopause madness or a midlife reawakening, call it what you will, I just woke up one day and thought, 'This is not how I want the rest of my life to play out.' My relationship was joyless; my husband systematically shut down my needs. I felt both suffocated and inexplicably lonely. I decided I'd rather be lonely on my own than lonely living with someone I no longer loved. So that was that. I'm now living on my own and the least lonely I've ever been.

Let's make this all about you

Chances are by now you've become pretty adept at single-handedly juggling a truckload of life tasks and responsibilities all at once. But it's impossible to keep all those plates spinning while simultaneously trying to deal with haywire hormones. Something has to give, and that something is you. You have to give yourself permission to be what we jokingly call selfish, but it is actually more like self-preservation. Sometimes we need reminding that it's ok to reclaim some space in our lives just for ourselves. There's a common refrain that says you can't look after everyone else if you're not looking after yourself. Well, quite frankly, screw everyone else. Our viewpoint is that you need to look after yourself for the sheer joy of finally spending some quality time with yourself, on your terms.

Get to know your new perimenopausal self. This is a whole new chapter, which can feel discombobulating. But do it for yourself. No one else. This is sometimes easier said than done. Our number one tip? Start saying 'no' more, albeit with kindness and respect. But a firm 'no' nonetheless. 'No,

I won't be able to make it.' 'I'm going to have to say no this time I'm afraid.' 'Unfortunately no, that isn't possible right now.' Try it. Not only is it liberating; it gives you back energy, time and focus that are much needed right now. Who knows, maybe you can make yourself more available when your hormones are back under control – if you choose to. But for now, don't be afraid to add 'no' to your lexicon and let it trip off your tongue freely. It's utterly freeing to put an end to patterns, relationships and procedures that no longer fit us. We're evolving, developing, growing. It's normal, natural and understandable. In many ways this brings us back to the perimenopause-as-reverse-puberty idea that we touched on earlier. Teenagers don't think twice about creating new boundaries for themselves, because they don't have a 'set' way of thinking. Likewise, perimenopausal women are dismantling the accepted norms of behaviour and starting to think a lot more for themselves.

Write here, write now

If talking feels too much for you right now, writing stuff down (journalling) can feel immensely unburdening. Getting thoughts out of your head and on to paper can also help you make sense of what you're feeling. This is especially helpful when your brain feels overwhelmed and disordered. There's no right or wrong way to go about journalling; it's a very personal thing. If you've never done it before, here are some tips to get you started.

»   Get a notebook and a pen and designate a place for them (we like the bedside table), both as a reminder but also to encourage the practice to become a habit.

» Spend anything from a couple of minutes to half an hour on it every day – there are no rules.

» Don't worry about ordering your thoughts; just get your words out on to the paper.

» Write for yourself, no one else is going to read this.

» Include doodles, pictures, diagrams, bullet points, lists and scribbles.

» We like to end with three positives or things we're grateful for to sign off.

Stay connected

There are lots of other ways to enter into a conversation about perimenopause:

» Try setting up a WhatsApp group with friends. You can keep it small or invite friends of friends and/or work colleagues in.

» Look for Facebook communities that appeal to you. There are lots of perimenopause and menopause ones.

» The Latte Lounge is a virtual coffee shop aimed at women over 40. It has over 20,000 members globally and is somewhere you can chat, ask questions, share tips and swap news.

» menopausecafe.net organise meet-ups across the world. It's open to all genders and all ages.

» If you prefer listening rather than contributing, there are lots of podcasts on offer. We like The Shift, Postcards from Midlife and The Midpoint with Gabby Logan (which the midlife men in your life may enjoy too).

The bottom line

» Don't underestimate mental health issues: during perimenopause, they can be just as prevalent and debilitating as physical symptoms.

» Understand your hormones: the decline in oestrogen during perimenopause can bring about emotions including sadness, dissatisfaction and despair. Sometimes, these can be diagnosed as menopausal mood disorder (MMD).

» Make the distinction: between MMD and other mental health issues, including depression and anxiety.

» Get the right support: options include lifestyle alterations, therapy and medication. Never suffer in silence because help is always available.

» Reach out to loved ones: some people in your life might not recognise what you're going through. Don't be afraid to spell it out.

» Take a deep breath: before making any big life decisions, get your hormones on an even keel. Then you'll know if you truly want to make that change, or if it's your hormones dictating the state of play.

» Journal: if a conversation is hard for you to engage in right now, think about writing it in a letter or setting your thoughts down in a journal

» Reclaim vital time for yourself: start saying 'no' more.

PART 2
Life

CHAPTER 7

Let's Talk About Sex

Self-love comes in many forms and sex and intimacy is another area to employ it. Allow your mind to open.

We live in a society where sex is often a taboo subject – you might feel reluctant to talk to your closest friends about it and bury your head in the sand rather than addressing sexual difficulties with your partner. But sex is too important to our health and wellbeing to ignore, so in this chapter we'll talk about how to navigate the emotional and physical minefield of getting intimate in perimenopause and beyond. Not least because orgasms are, quite simply, brilliant for your health. If we could prescribe them, we would!

In our teens and 20s, we think about people in their 40s or 50s having sex and it seems gross and unthinkable. Fast-forward 25 years and we realise we still want to be sexual and vivacious, but our sex lives *are* far more nuanced and complicated than we'd ever imagined back in the hedonistic days of our youth.

A loss of libido or sex drive and desire can affect one third of women at some point in their lives, and during perimenopause can be all the more common due to diminishing hormones. You may feel that you're the only one it's happening to – but remember you're not! It doesn't bother some women or affect their relationship, while for others it can be quite distressing and persistent – medically it is known as Hypoactive Sexual Desire Disorder (HSDD).

Often it's the hormonal and biological changes that characterise perimenopause that begin to make us feel disconnected from who we used to be and contribute to our libido taking a dip. We become tired, irritable and feel unsettled by our changing appearance and then there are the other physical challenges that are worsened by the perimenopause, such as vaginal dryness and discomfort, or even pain, during sex. On top of all this, there's the 'life stuff' – families, friends, careers, children and households to manage. It's hardly surprising to find 51 per cent of women say the menopause affected their sex lives, while 40 per cent admitted that they didn't feel as sexy since experiencing the menopause, describing sex with their partners as 'duty' or 'mercy' sex.

Sex is good for you

The phrase 'use it or lose it' definitely applies to our vaginas. If we don't use them, we'll notice our vaginal health declines. Doctors use the term 'genitourinary syndrome of menopause' (GSM) to describe the symptoms that can occur during perimenopause. This means the vagina can atrophy (shrink), become drier and even shorten in length. There is also 'clitoral atrophy' – when the clitoris shrinks – and, considering it's the part of our body solely dedicated to our pleasure, it's essential to sexual satisfaction.

Our pelvic floor health can also be affected by perimenopausal hormone decline (see page 185). A 'dragging' sensation, or a feeling of heaviness in the vagina, is due to the impact of decreasing oestrogen. Externally, too, the labia, vulva and the skin around the vagina becomes crepier and less plump. As the vaginal environment becomes more alkaline, there is an increased risk of urinary tract infections and yeast infections, like thrush.

Localised oestrogen (see box) can tackle some of the physical vaginal symptoms, but simply having more sex helps too, as well as improving your mental health and wellbeing. And, while having sex is not quite 'exercise', you can still get a sweat on! The good news is that you don't have to be having partnered sex, which may be a first for many women – a new revelation and a new sensation, so go on give it a go (see page 116)!

Orgasms are good for us – they promote positive physical and emotional wellbeing, boosting our circulation and increasing blood supply to the vagina, which helps promote vaginal cell multiplication, improves lubrication, and enhances the plumpness, 'springiness' and length of the vagina. Orgasms are also positive for our mental health; when you have one, your brain produces those happy hormones – serotonin, dopamine and noradrenaline – as well as the 'love' hormone, oxytocin, the release of which makes us feel warm and glowing.

Self-love comes in many forms and sex and intimacy is another area to employ it. Allow your mind to open!

Causes of low sex drive

There are many factors that can contribute to a lower libido:

» Hormonal changes: a drop in oestrogen and testosterone levels
» Physical causes: pain during sex, vulvo-vaginal atrophy
» Medical conditions: diabetes, arthritis, obesity, neurological diseases, cardiovascular disease
» Relationship/communication breakdown: unresolved issues, trust issues
» Low self-esteem
» Low body confidence
» Depression
» History of abuse
» Fatigue, stress and anxiety
» Certain medications, e.g. some antidepressants
» Surgery: this can affect your perception of your body and lower your self-esteem
» Lifestyle: excess alcohol consumption and smoking, which can reduce blood flow and dull arousal

Medical treatments

The physical changes of vaginal dryness, which can make sex feel uncomfortable or even downright painful, can often be treated with a good lubricant, or with prescribed treatments such as HRT, and vulvo-vaginal oestrogen creams and pessaries. Vaginal laser treatment (see page 83) may also help to improve the libido. Women who take testosterone (see page 60) often report an increase in their mood, energy, muscle strength, stamina and libido and it is a recommended treatment in the NICE guidelines for treatment of HSDD (see page 111).

Get your mojo back or not

There are many reasons why we might have a reduced libido (see box), but when we really unpick the complex dynamics around why we have the amount of sex we do, a lot comes down to you as a woman and how confident you feel in your maturing body and mind. First, you may need to fall back in love with yourself. It can be hard to regain lost confidence and surmount the mental hurdle in your brain that has stopped you seeing yourself as a sexual person. So how can you bring sexy back?

Well, first you need to be a little bit selfish for what might be the first time in many decades and get back in touch with who you are. What is your identity? Have you slipped into being defined by what you are to other people: a mother, wife, daughter, friend, boss or colleague?

The first step to regaining your confidence – to remembering who *you* are – is doing something for yourself. We hereby give you permission to be selfish, which isn't easy when you've spent most of your life as a giver and people pleaser. I hope hearing this helps you realise taking time to do something *you* want to do doesn't make you a bad partner, mother or employee.

Invest in yourself by doing one or two of these feel-good hacks and see if they help you to feel better connected to what brings you joy.

» Listen to your favourite music.
» Go for a bike ride or a country drive.
» Have a beauty treatment.
» Go to the cinema on your own.
» Visit a gallery or museum.
» Start a journal.
» Tune into a podcast.
» Read (or try an audio book), maybe while going for a walk or soaking in the bath (the perfect place to multitask).
» Relax in the garden or somewhere else in nature.
» Wear no underwear – it's amazing how it can make you feel mischievous and naughty, even more so if you casually drop it into a conversation with your partner.
» Indulge in some retail therapy.
» Dig out that bright coloured lipstick that you haven't been bold enough to wear.
» Actually phone someone who you've not spoken to in a while.
» Spend some time in the kitchen making a delicious cake or something nourishing for the week ahead.
» Paint, draw, write a poem; bring out your creative side.
» Do a jigsaw puzzle – the perfect mindful activity.

We're all different, so just think back to the things that used to 'relight your fire'. What are the things you enjoy or would like to try out? Dare yourself. The idea is to do little things that remind you of who you are, where you come from and what you've achieved. They will serve to reconnect you with what brings you pleasure.

Masturbation: 'self-love'

Self-stimulation, or masturbation, is a taboo subject. Even women who partake in it and get a lot out of it don't usually want to talk about it. We need to break that stigma down so that women feel comfortable discovering – and rediscovering – their own bodies. It's one of the healthiest way to practise self-love because of the myriad of health benefits of orgasms.

Your perimenopausal sexual journey might involve putting sex with your partner on hold for a few months while you relearn how to enjoy the feelings and sensations your body can give you. If you feel like it's a necessary part of your sexual reawakening, prioritise masturbation over partnered sex. Giving things a go on your own before doing them with somebody else will mean you go into sex with more confidence. For now, it's time to get back in touch with yourself – literally. We believe practising makes us feel more confident in whatever we're about to embark on – whether that's singing a song on stage, giving a work presentation, or, yes, getting back into the sexual swing of things with a partner – which is why, either way, it's key that masturbation precedes partnered sex. How are you supposed to explain what you want if you don't know yourself?

First of all, pick up a mirror and have a look down there. When was the last time you properly connected with what your vulva and vagina looks like? Maybe you've never done it. But they're part of your body, so get acquainted with them.

Start by finding some space where you can feel relaxed, knowing you won't be interrupted. Get familiar with your body, maybe stand in front of the mirror, take it all in. Start by stroking your skin on your neck, putting your fingers through your hair and keep your focus on you. How does it feel? Stroke your shoulders, taking in the sensation of your skin being stroked; look at your breasts, gently stroke them, working your way around one breast then the other and gently brushing across your nipples, lightly and increasing in intensity. Allow yourself to relax, to concentrate on the sensations in your body, and how it makes you feel. Take it at your pace. Allow your fingers to glide down to between your legs, stroking between the lips of your vulva and touch your clitoris. Stroke your legs and inner thighs. Do as much or as little as you feel comfortable and maybe build upon it each time. Remember, orgasms are good for your health!

Your self-stimulation toolkit

Lubrication: make life a little easier and less stressful by applying some lube – choose oil-based if you are using sex toys. Knowing that you're going to be wet reduces some anticipatory anxiety, and anxiety itself takes the fun away and can reduce your own natural lubrication.

Vibrators come in various shapes and sizes. You don't need to insert it fully; press it not only against your clitoris but also your nipples and feel your body awake from the vibrations. You can always upscale later once you get comfortable and into a rhythm.

Porn: most porn still presents women in a derogatory light, so patients are often surprised when it gets recommended as part of their self-stimulation ritual, but we're not talking about degrading, misogynistic porn. Ethical porn, which is often made by women for women, is available – try Erika Lust's XConfessions, which shows erotic films based on real life scenarios; Bellesa, where women's pleasure is prioritised; or Pink Label TV, which streams feminist, queer, BIPOC and non-binary films.

Erotic audio: gentler – yet no less erotic – readings or audio recordings are available on apps like Ferly and Dipsea.

Clit lit: if you get off on erotic literature rather than visuals, check out Frolic Me which is female-friendly, free to read and features stories written by leading edge porn writers.

Sex with your partner

Communicating with your partner as you work to regain your confidence in and outside of the bedroom is so important. But brushing the 'whole sex thing' under the rug is incredibly common, particularly in a long-term relationship, not least because you many not want to offend your partner or make him feel rejected. Rather than tackle these difficulties, it's easy to slip into a friendship-relationship and feel happy, for a while, in that place. But in the long-term, it's much healthier to get how you're feeling out in the open. Talking about it is like lifting the lid off a pressure cooker: it'll allow some of the anxiety and, yes, pressure, to dissipate.

Countless relationship breakdowns and divorces happen in this trench because the pressures of modern life make prioritising sex even more difficult: you might both be so busy that you're like ships that pass in the night. Even though you're physically seeing each other, you're not really *seeing* the other person or spending that much quality time with them.

Making the time to talk to your partner about your sex life is important – you're not just going to jump straight into bed together if you haven't had sex in a while or you're not in the right headspace. How you go about it will be personal to you, but here are some ideas ... Try doing something relaxing to lower your inhibitions before you have the chat.

If you prefer not to have direct eye contact, you may prefer to talk while you're walking or driving side by side. Some people find it easier to write things down. One woman told me that she and her partner sat on the sofa next to each and wrote messages in their iPhone notes app about how they were respectively dealing with the sexual stalemate they'd found themselves in. Do whatever works best for you.

A good starting point is to explain how your perimenopausal symptoms have been making you feel; that your loss of libido – as well as irritability, sensitivity, anger and fatigue – are caused by hormonal changes. Make it clear: 'It's not that I don't love or care about you; it's that my hormones are making me feel like I'm not myself right now.' All partners require affirmation in a relationship – everybody needs to feel important and loved – so communicating you're not rejecting your partner is an important aspect of this journey.

Give your partner time to take everything in – and I'm not just talking about men. If your partner is a younger woman, she may struggle to understand what you're going through because she's not where you are yet. In fairness, you may only just be getting to grips with the symptoms yourself.

After having the chat, it's unlikely you'll have sex that night, but expressing your feelings – and your boundaries – will help your partner understand where they stand. If you're not ready to restart the sexual side of your relationship yet, say, 'I really want to focus on getting myself back into a better place, so I just need some time to do that.'

Where you take it from there is personal to you both as a couple. You might, for example, decide to take penetrative sex off the agenda for a month, and focus more on kissing, cuddling and foreplay. You may want to work on rediscovering your body and increasing your confidence. When you do feel like having sex again, a great way in is to share some of the things you most enjoyed from the 'self-stimulation toolkit' (see page 117). Could you watch porn together? Or use a sex toy? Bring the things that help you into your relationship with your partner and you'll likely find they enhance your sexual connection, developing it into an exciting new phase.

Most importantly, don't expect things to be resolved overnight and keep talking and communicating and taking your partner's feelings into account. Although it may feel like it at times, your perimenopausal journey isn't just yours; it also belongs to your partner and everybody else around you, so be mindful of their feelings, too.

It may be that you can't resolve the sexual stalemate yourselves. In this case, you might want to consider seeing a sex therapist – having a third person involved to facilitate the conversation and suggest things you can try can help.

Dave's story

My partner Emma's second cancer diagnosis and the maintenance chemo she was on meant that she'd been thrown into an early menopause. A monthly injection of a hormone therapy called Zoladex to ensure her ovaries stopped making oestrogen was a double whammy.

We quickly went from being madly in love, beautiful lovemaking and falling asleep in each other's arms to feeling disconnected, low and irritable.

At first I felt upset, but in time that led to anger. I also felt rejected. I started to blame Em and reject her myself and we began to regularly fall out. I would hear her sobbing in the bedroom, but my own hurt and frustration stopped me from reaching out.

It wasn't until I went with Em to a hospital appointment that what she'd been going through really hit me. The consultant asked how she was coping with the side-effects of treatment, and listened sympathetically as she admitted she was struggling. I felt mortified. How could I have been so insensitive? Why was I so selfish?

I held her hand in the car on the way home and that night at bedtime I held her tight and told her how sorry I was. I told her how much I loved her and she cried. She said she'd felt confused and lost and scared because she thought she would lose me.

The most important thing I learned from this was I should have put my feelings aside and asked questions. What she needed was sensitivity, unconditional love, understanding and lots of reassurance.

Now every three weeks, and always a couple of days after the Zoladex injection, we actually giggle at the mood change and give each other a huge hug and remind ourselves it's hard for both of us.

Jade's story

I'd always really enjoyed sex, then just went off it. I was 46 and my boyfriend, who was 10 years younger, always seemed up for it so I would make some excuses, that I was tired or had to get up early the next day. Sometimes I just went through the motions. As I felt so dry, sex felt uncomfortable.

I would secretly go into the bathroom to apply lube as I didn't want my boyfriend to think that I wasn't turned on.

Eventually I went to my doctor who reassured me that the vaginal dryness was a common perimenopausal symptom and prescribed topical oestrogen. She also talked to me about how I was feeling. I said I wasn't feeling confident in myself and was nervous that sex would be uncomfortable. I was taken aback when she recommended a bit of self-love! She suggested that I go and watch some porn and invest in a slimline vibrator, which I did. I took it at my own pace and noticed how my body responded. This made me feel more confident about having and enjoying sex with my boyfriend – it's certainly true that the more you do it, the more you want it and the better you feel!

The bottom line

» Hormonal changes can cause a double whammy – physical changes to your vagina and a loss of interest in sex.

» Sex is good for you: not having it – specifically, not having orgasms – can worsen your physical symptoms and mean you don't benefit from the emotional highs that pleasure can bring.

» Rebuild your confidence by doing something that's just for you. Remember, buy the shoes, not the frying pan.

» Masturbate: there's no shame in it – in fact, touching yourself can help you reconnect to what makes you feel good and reawaken your sexual side.

» Talk about it: remember it's normal if your feelings around sex have changed. Communicating your feelings to your partner will work wonders for the long-term health of your relationship, even if you don't jump into bed again straight away. Consider seeing a sex therapist if you need to.

CHAPTER 8

Sleep Smarter

A healthy perimenopause starts in bed.

For many women, poor-quality sleep is the first sign that perimenopause is starting to kick in. More often than not, sleep disruption is put down to stress, family issues or the sheer overwhelm that comes with midlife. Not many women make the hormone connection. Progesterone is known for its calming, melatonin-producing qualities, so when levels drop many women experience insomnia-related issues. Many women find their sleep improves dramatically when hormone levels are brought back in line. But there are many more natural solutions – from quietening down a snoring partner to dietary changes. Modern life coupled with perimenopause problems can make sleep elusive, but as you'll see throughout this chapter, it's worth working on.

None of us who have had it, need to be told how crippling insomnia can be: how it affects mood, performance at work, energy levels, concentration and even how we look. Everything feels worse after a restless night. Plus, worrying about sleep can easily cross over into obsession, often fuelled by gadgets and digital trackers – a phenomenon so prevalent it has a name: orthosomnia. Ever lay in bed wide awake, trying to put your finger on why it is you can't sleep? The answer, as always, is multi-factorial:

» Progesterone plays a role in melatonin production, which helps you fall asleep and stay asleep. Reduced levels of progesterone during perimenopause leads to less sleep.
» Low levels of oestrogen can cause disruptive symptoms, not least night sweats.
» Melatonin, the sleep-signalling hormone, decreases as we age.
» Anxiety and overwhelm from the pressures of everyday life.
» Joint pain.
» Bladder issues/getting up to go to the toilet.
» Medical conditions like hyperthyroidism, arthritis and tinnitus.
» Sleep apnoea.
» Alcohol (increases night sweats, anxiety, palpitations).
» Interruptions from children.
» Keto/very low-carb diet (carbs help calm the nervous system).
» A snoring partner.
» Prescription medication (beta blockers and blood pressure medication, antidepressants, corticosteroids).
» Heartburn.
» Restless leg syndrome.
» Low iron.

It might sound like an exhaustive list but there are ways to fix it, and we're here to help.

How much sleep do you need?

Not everyone needs the often quoted eight hours of sleep a night; some people function perfectly well on seven, while others might need closer to nine. It's also worth remembering that sleeping requirements change and some women find that, as they age, they need less sleep. As with so many other aspects of health, it really is individual so try to focus on what works for you, rather than getting alarmed that you're not meeting the population level quotas that are often mentioned in research.

The best way to gauge whether you are getting enough sleep is to spend a week noting down how much sleep you think you're getting (no gadgets required) and how you feel the next day. Do you need an alarm clock to wake you up? Are you heavily reliant on caffeine? Do you wake feeling refreshed? Quality is just as important as quantity. Ideally, we want to be waking no more than once a night, to be asleep around 85 per cent of the time we're in bed (i.e. not taking hours to drift off and not staring at the ceiling as dawn breaks) and to be getting plenty of deep, uninterrupted sleep. It is easy for us to say, but please try not to stress over exact numbers as it's counterproductive – we know many clients who have become unhealthily obsessed with the stats from their gadgets that measure sleep, and have actually fared far better in the sleep stakes once they ditched it.

Increase your appetite for sleep

The fundamental key to a good night's sleep is to build up your appetite for it throughout the day. As soon as you wake up, you're looking to insert as many drivers as you can that increase the need for sleep at bedtime. These include:

» Exposure to early morning daylight (which helps set your body clock)
» Exercise
» The amount of time you've been awake
» Fresh air

Things that can hinder the drive to sleep:

» Naps, particularly long ones taken later in the day
» Sleeping in at the weekend
» Going to bed earlier than usual
» Too much caffeine
» Stress (cortisol)

Dim your evenings, brighten your days

The first light we are exposed to in the morning plays a key role in how alert we feel during the day and how soundly we sleep at night. Getting exposure to daylight as soon as you can after waking – and getting outside as much as possible in the first half of the day – will help set your wake-sleep cycle for the next 24 hours. This might mean taking a work call outside rather than at your desk, exercising in a park instead of in a gym, or having your morning cuppa in the garden or, at the very least, sitting next to a naturally well-lit window.

And come evening, you need to flip this on its head. Melatonin is secreted as darkness falls. It's basically nature's way of signalling sleep is coming and we need to start winding down. Unhelpfully, our ability to produce melatonin decreases as we age (it's also influenced by oestrogen and progesterone, which compounds the problem as hormone levels decrease during perimenopause) so we need to be scrupulous in our attempts to maximise it. We can help by turning off overhead lights, lighting candles, using dim table lamps and avoiding blue light from handheld devices.

Medical treatments

Disrupted sleep is one of the first symptoms to improve with hormone replacement therapy (HRT) (see Chapter 4). Many studies have consistently shown HRT's positive effects on sleep, particularly in women who have vasomotor symptoms such as hot flushes and night sweats.

Progesterone plays a key role for its sleep-inducing effect and has been linked with increased non-REM stage 3 sleep, in other words deep sleep. Even if you don't need progesterone as part of your HRT prescription, perhaps because you've had a hysterectomy, it's possible to take micronised progesterone for its beneficial effect on sleep.

If you think you're suffering from a disorder such as sleep apnoea, where the walls of the throat relax and narrow during sleep, interrupting normal breathing, seek advice from your doctor or a sleep specialist. It's more common in women who are overweight or obese and, as we know, this is a time of life when our weight creeps up. Also, oestrogen and progesterone maintain the integrity of the airways, so as levels decline, incidences of sleep apnoea increase.

Nothing changes if nothing changes

How many times have you been told that blue light from screens interrupts sleep signals and causes fragmented rest? Yet how often are you still on your phone at 11pm for one last scroll, tweet, double tap, inbox refresh? Thought so. Below, we will discuss some sleep strategies. Try to look at the following R.E.S.T. strategies – Routine, Environment, Sleep aids, Timing – with fresh eyes. Choose three or four that you can actively put in place from tonight for a minimum of one month.

Even if you feel they're not making a difference, stick with them and come back to choose a couple more when the four weeks is up. Be proactive. You don't get change without change.

Routine

Your body clock loves routine, so try to go to bed and wake up at the same time each day, even at weekends. Bear in mind it might take a few weeks or longer to establish and stick to your new set times, so don't give up. Habits take a while to form, but once set aren't going anywhere.

Aim to finish your last meal around three hours before bedtime. To help maintain good blood-sugar balance (see page 140) throughout the night, you need to find the sweet spot between being neither hungry nor full. If you need a light snack, go for it, but stay away from high-sugar foods and drinks. A snack such as an oat cake with peanut butter works well.

Avoid stimulants – sugar, smoking, caffeine and alcohol – before bed, no matter how tempting. Alcohol might help you nod off because it's a sedative, but it negatively impacts your REM sleep (which helps with mood and memory) and makes the rest of your sleep much more fragmented, so you wake early and unrefreshed. It also raises your core body temperature (hello night sweats) and increases your resting heart rate.

Try not to drink too much liquid after 7pm to prevent having to get up in the night to go to the toilet.

Switch your devices to come on to night mode automatically from 7pm. The blue light emitted from them confuses the brain into thinking it's daytime and stops the secretion of melatonin. In one study, staring at a screen before bed for an hour blocked melatonin by 50 per cent and shortened melatonin duration by 90 minutes. Alternatively, install f.lux on all devices, which adjusts your screen colour, depending on the time of the day.

Don't nap after 3pm, and keep any naps to 20 minutes max. While napping can help with short-term memory and concentration, as mentioned earlier it may well block sleep appetite.

Sleep experts recommend that if you wake during the night and can't get back to sleep, it is better to get up and do something else: reading seems to work well. Avoid looking on your phone or other gadgets and keep the lights low.

Environment

Your body needs to drop its core temperature by about one degree to initiate sleep and to stay asleep throughout the night. The optimal bedroom temperature is therefore a cool 18°C. Turn radiators off, keep windows open in the run up to bedtime or invest in a fan. Having a bath can induce sleepiness because your body temperature drops after getting out of the warm water. Use Epsom salts in your bath (buy bulk in 5/10/20kg bags online) to absorb calming magnesium (see page 139) through your skin.

Dim the lights in the evening to help signal the release of melatonin, the sleep hormone. When existing bulbs run out in lamps, consider replacing them with red incandescent light bulbs.

Keep your bedroom dark: invest in blackout blinds or add blackout material to your existing curtains. If that's not possible, try wearing an eye mask.

Ear plugs can be helpful if noise is an issue where you live or you're a light sleeper. Make sure you keep them clean or replace them regularly if they're disposable.

De-clutter your bedroom so it's a haven of tranquility: a calm room equals calm mind.

Keep gadgets out of the bedroom if possible. They can lengthen the time it takes you to drop off, encourage you to wake in the middle of the night for a quick scroll, and often cause an onslaught of stress if they're the first thing you look at on waking.

Solutions for snoring partners

It's hard to think of anything more palpitation-inducing than lying next to a snoring partner while you're trying to drift off. We know many relation-ships have been saved by a strategic move into the spare room. If that's not possible – and an elbow in the side is no longer cutting it – all is not lost. We asked our followers on social media for their best snoring hacks. Here are a few options to try:

» Talk to a dentist about fitting a mandibular repositioning device – a made-to-measure anti-snoring mouth guard. If that's out of your budget, try a cheaper online option. Just search for 'anti-snoring mouthpiece'.
» Nose vent – opens up nostrils and improves air flow.
» Mouth taping – this thin medical tape is used to tape the mouth shut and encourage (quieter) nose breathing. Eventually this should become second nature, with no need for

taping. Caution: it is not advisable for anyone with low blood pressure, severe nasal breathing or heart health problems.

» Snoring ring – worn on the little finger, this is said to work through acupressure. There are mixed reviews of this, if we're honest, and it is not exactly grounded in science, but it is a cheap experiment (most online are under a tenner) if you want to try it.

» Anti-snoring pillow – encourages the sleeper to stay on their side, thereby reducing the likelihood of snoring.

» CPAP machine – if all else fails, try this ventilator that is worn over the nose and mouth and pushes air into the lungs to facilitate breathing. We had a client who swears this saved her marriage. It's not cheap and it's certainly not a turn-on, but if it means a decent night's sleep, it might just be worth the investment.

Sleep aids

Reusable cooling pads: place these under your sheet or inside your pillowcase if you suffer from night sweats. They're effective on their own, but you can give them even more cool factor by leaving them in the fridge or freezer for a couple of hours (a frozen 'hot' water bottle works well too). If you share a bed, buy a single-sized pad to avoid interfering with your partner's sleep.

Specialist bedding: natural fibre bedsheets and light-weight night clothes made from sweat-wicking fabrics like bamboo can help if you have night sweats. Be careful, though, as there are lots of hot-flush-friendly clothing companies making all sorts of wild claims about their 'nanotechnology'; most are unfounded and the products eye-wateringly expensive. One thing you can do is remove mattress toppers as they can trap heat, and be aware that memory foam is also known for raising temperatures. If you share a bed, it can be helpful to buy two single duvets rather than sharing one large one. Having your own duvet allows you to regulate your temperature much more easily.

SAD lamp: this lamp mimics natural daylight and is particularly effective in winter. A built-in wake-up function encourages you to start the day gradually rather than with the jarring sound of an alarm.

Light-blocking glasses: try wearing a pair of amber-lensed blue-light-blocking glasses in the afternoon if much of your day is spent in front of a screen. In a 2009 randomised trial, wearers experienced 'significant improvement' in sleep.

Aromatherapy products: although there's no solid science behind aromatherapy, pillow sprays and essential oils can be a valuable part of a wind-down routine.

Weighted blankets: as well as reducing the amount you move around in bed, the hug-like pressure that these blankets exert is said to be reassuring, thereby reducing anxiety. This was backed up by a study in *Occupational Therapy and Mental Health* that found 63 per cent of adults reported lower anxiety after sleeping with a 14kg blanket. They are expensive, but some brands offer 100-day trials with a full money-back guarantee. If you suffer from night sweats, make sure you look out for cooling varieties that are designed to maximise airflow and are made from breathable material.

Mindful breathing

To help you relax at bedtime or during the night, try the 3–4–5 breath. Breathe in through your nose for a count of 3 seconds, hold for 4 seconds, breathe out through your mouth for 5 seconds. Repeat for as many cycles as needed. The longer out-breath helps the calming aspect of your nervous system kick in and is really useful any time you feel anxiety levels rise.

You can also find guided mindfulness meditations on apps like Headspace, Calm or Insight Timer.

Timing

Avoid anything too adrenaline-boosting before bedtime – for example, watching a horror movie and talking about stressful topics before bed. Ideally, leave at least a four-hour gap between exercising and bedtime, as it raises your core temperature and elevates cortisol, neither of which are conducive to gentle drifting off to sleep.

As our brains are kept busy all day, it's not surprising we start playing things over and over in our mind as soon as we are lying in bed. To counteract this, schedule 15 minutes of 'worry time' in the run up to bed. Write to-do lists or jot down any thoughts or problems that might preoccupy you during the night. Often, what feels overwhelming bouncing around in your mind can look far less daunting when put down on paper. One pilot study showed keeping a journal helped participants fall asleep more quickly and another showed the benefits of writing a to-do list before hitting the hay. Keep a journal and pen next to your bed to remind you to get into the habit.

Sleep and smartphones do not make good bedfellows. Try to impose a rule that you don't look at your phone after 9pm, or even better, keep it out of the bedroom completely. If you usually use it to wake you up, invest in an old-fashioned (non-ticking) alarm clock or a SAD lamp (see page 133).

If you *have* to scroll while you're in bed, best make it something soothing. The Calm app has a great resource called *Sleep Stories* read in the soporific tones of Matthew McConaughey, Harry Styles and Stephen Fry. Sign up for the free 7-day trial before you commit.

CBT-I

Cognitive Behavioural Therapy for Insomnia (CBT-I) is an evidence-based approach and is the first-line therapy (before sleeping pills, which have lots of side-effects) for ongoing sleep issues. Talk to your doctor about finding a local practitioner or try an online course like Sleepio, which teaches you long-term cognitive and sleep-behaviour techniques. Many participants see benefits within weeks, or even days, and the programme has been shown to be just as effective as seeing a therapist face to face.

Eat to sleep

There isn't a magic food that sends you off to never-never land, but foods that contain tryptophan might help bring on a peaceful slumber. Tryptophan is an amino acid that helps stimulate the production of serotonin and sleep-promoting melatonin – it's said to be partly why we all fall asleep on the sofa after a tryptophan-rich turkey dinner at Christmas.

Tryptophan food sources include:

» Chicken
» Turkey
» Salmon
» Canned tuna
» Tofu
» Eggs
» Milk
» Greek yoghurt
» Nuts and seeds
» Chickpeas
» Bananas
» Oats
» Broccoli

To increase the likelihood of these foods making you feel sleepy, pair a tryptophan protein source with a carbohydrate before bed: good combinations include Greek yoghurt with banana, apple with almonds, or tuna with broccoli and chickpeas.

Pay attention to the amount of B vitamins you're getting, especially B6 (found in chicken, turkey, peanuts, oats, bananas, milk and fortified cereals) and B12 (mainly found in animal products like meat, fish and dairy). These, together with magnesium (found in green leafy vegetables, such as spinach and kale), help to increase GABA – a neurotransmitter known for its calming qualities – and also play a role in treating PMS and low mood.

You should be able to get all the B6 you need from your diet, but if you're worried your nutrition is sub-par and you want to supplement, talk to a healthcare practitioner first, especially as large doses (in excess of 100mg) taken long-term (more than a year) can cause permanent peripheral neuropathy (numbness) in your arms and legs. Interestingly, you may find B6 makes your dreams more vivid and easier to recall. If vegan or vegetarian, you should be supplementing daily with 10mg of B12 as standard (for more info and dosage details, see page 255).

Caffeine

The chemical adenosine tells us when we're sleepy and it naturally builds up over the course of the day. Caffeine blocks it, which is why so many of us rely on coffee to prop us up when we're flagging in that 2–4pm window. Caffeine affects us all differently, mainly due to genetics, but the general rule is not to exceed 400mg a day.

Caffeine has a half-life of six hours (or more) and a quarter life of 12 hours, so that means if you're having a coffee at noon, a quarter of it is still in your bloodstream at midnight. Caffeine-loving insomniacs won't appreciate this, but if you're having issues with sleep it might be worth avoiding caffeine after breakfast. Try it for four weeks to see if it helps. Remember caffeine isn't only found in tea and coffee (see box), so be aware of other sources, especially if you're sensitive to caffeine.

If you're flagging in the afternoon, instead of having a double shot espresso, try getting up and walking around or going outside. It's a surprisingly effective way of jolting yourself out of a lull.

For later in the day, many women find 'sleepy' teas a soothing alternative – look for ingredients like valerian root, passionflower, lavender, lemon balm and chamomile – but try to finish taking on fluids by 7pm.

Sources of caffeine

Use this table to work out your daily caffeine consumption.

	Average caffeine content (mg)
Brewed coffee (240ml)	135
Instant coffee (240ml)	95
Decaf coffee (240ml)	5
Espresso (60ml)	80
Latte/Cappuccino/ Macchiato (240ml)	80
Black tea (240ml)	50
Green tea (240ml)	45
Dark chocolate 70% (50g)	40
Cola (330ml)	40
Energy drink (500ml)	160
Cold and flu medication	Ranges from 25–50mg per dose (check label)

Supplements

Before you start cleaning up the vitamin aisle, it's advisable to work on getting all the other sleep foundations in place. Lifestyle changes will yield better results than capsules, which aren't the quick fix people hope for. It's remarkable how often we see women in clinic who are on the floor with tiredness and rattling with pills, but who flat out refuse to knock their wine habit on the head. That said, here are a few supplements you might want to add to your super sleep strategy, but seriously, work on the alcohol and caffeine first!

Melatonin: unlike in the USA, melatonin can't be bought over the counter in the UK (some people stock up when they go on holiday), but it can be prescribed by your doctor. There isn't a huge amount of evidence linking melatonin in supplement form to long-lasting good sleep. For most people it only works as a temporary fix for jet lag, but it might be something to talk to your doctor about.

L-theanine: this has been linked with better sleep in people with anxiety. One study used 450–900mg daily for eight weeks.

Glycine: this has many roles in the body, one of which is making serotonin and melatonin that work to calm the brain. It has been linked with falling asleep faster and having better-quality sleep. Take 3g before bed.

Magnesium: as many as 7 out of 10 women in the UK are estimated to be deficient in magnesium. Low levels can impact sleep and a whole raft of related perimenopause symptoms, including anxiety, palpitations, restless legs and fatigue. Magnesium works by supporting GABA (which calms the brain), reducing glutamate (which stimulates the brain) and lowering the stress hormone cortisol. Try starting with 300mg magnesium glycinate, which combines the calming action of glycine, an hour before bed. You can build up your dose as needed but ask a professional for guidance.

Taurine: this works by calming GABA receptors. Interestingly it is often found in energy drinks to counteract the stimulating effects of caffeine. The therapeutic dose for sleep is 3g taken before bed.

Montmorency cherry (or tart cherry) juice: this contains tryptophan and melatonin and is often touted as a sleep aid, although robust research is scant. If you want to try for yourself, look for sugar-free versions and aim to take 300–400ml in the evening.

Why sugar and sleep don't mix

It's been a full-on day and to wind down you enjoy a few glasses of wine or a bar of chocolate in front of Netflix. You go to bed and fall asleep. But what goes up must come down, so after about 3–4 hours your raised blood-sugar levels (from the wine or chocolate) suddenly drop. Your body senses this and, in response, releases a surge of cortisol, which wakes you up (it's not called the fight-or-flight response for nothing). You wake with your heart pounding, feeling anxious and stressed. The cortisol stress response triggers a hot flush and palpitations. You lie in bed feeling sweaty and out of control, wondering what the hell is wrong with you. You get up, change your night clothes and maybe even your sheets. You return to bed with a racing mind and find it difficult to get back to sleep. Eventually you doze off only for your alarm to wake you an hour later. You haul yourself out of bed and somehow get through the next 12 hours. You arrive home exhausted. You cheer yourself up with a few glasses of wine, some chocolate and Netflix …

Blood-sugar regulation plays a crucial role in getting an uninterrupted night's sleep. It's something that crops up repeatedly, both in terms of addressing symptoms, but also for long-term health. For a list of strategies to manage blood-sugar levels, turn to page 163.

The bottom line

» Sleep enhances every system in your body. It's like a nocturnal salve that helps your organs grow, build, relax, repair and restore.

» Plot out a wind-down routine and try to stick to it as much as possible each night. This is especially important when it comes to the time you go to sleep and wake up. Try to stick to it even after a bad night's sleep and at weekends.

» Make sure you get a blast of daylight first thing in the morning to set your circadian 'clock' and dim the lights in the evening to help with melatonin production.

» Avoid having caffeine after breakfast if you're really struggling with your sleep.

» Tighten up your sleep hygiene: no screens before bed, avoid stimulants, have a warm bath, keep your room dark and cool.

» Try including some tryptophan-containing foods in your evening meal.

» Work on keeping your blood-sugar levels as stable as possible. This is important throughout the day but even more so in the evening.

CHAPTER 9

Working It Out

Don't underestimate the influence
work has on your sense of self.
Rather than quitting, improve your
working life by asking for what you
need.

*It's well known that being pregnant and starting a family
can adversely impact a woman's career. What's less
talked about, however, is how the perimenopause and its
symptoms can disrupt our working lives. From dealing with
memory lapses to asking for help, and even establishing a
menopause policy in your workplace, we'll cover it all in this
chapter.*

Here we are in the 21st century and it's shocking that equality in the workplace still has some way to go. The gender
pay gap nationally stands at 18.4 per cent for full-time
and part-time workers, according to the UK's Office for
National Statistics (ONS). According to the ONS, 47 per cent
of the working population are women – yes, almost half the

working population – and yet the gender pay gap is that high. Considering 70–80 per cent of all menopausal-aged women are in work and numbers are increasing, it's ever-more important that women's needs in the workplace are taken into consideration. We are an economic force to be reckoned with!

As almost half of all women aged 45–55 find it difficult to cope with work during the menopause transition, it's time to take women's health seriously.

Vanessa's story

I noticed my periods started to become a bit hit-and-miss when I was 44. I could cope with them, but I was struggling to deal with what had happened to my brain. My usual mental sharpness had deserted me, and my brain felt clouded and foggy. I couldn't think clearly.

At the time, I was working at a magazine in a role I adored and had a team of young, brilliant women climbing the ladder underneath me, but I felt like I couldn't keep up with the pace.

I was losing confidence fast, making mistakes far more regularly than before and, on top of that, I was sleeping badly, which made me short-tempered and irritable. I wondered if I was becoming one of those grumpy 'middle aged' women.

After three years battling with these symptoms, I decided to take a career break. I made the decision after giving a terrible presentation at work. The words weren't flowing and I felt like I was frantically paddling to keep my head above water. I managed to get through it and explain it away with a feigned headache, but I knew I couldn't continue and didn't want to keep feeling pressure in this way. Giving up my salary put pressure on my family's finances and meant

I relinquished my financial independence, but I didn't feel like I had a choice.

Three years later, I went back to work at the same magazine as a freelancer. My supervisor was a woman who, years earlier, I'd trained. I felt embarrassed and also a failure. I'm now on HRT and have overhauled my lifestyle; drinking less, eating better and taking pride in who I am. I'm back to feeling like the sharp, confident woman I was and can't help but think that if that had happened five years ago, I might still be thriving in the old job I loved. Nevertheless, I now have the confidence to apply for more senior positions and have embraced my newfound freedom as a freelancer and have the confidence to pitch for work.

Were it not for Vanessa's crippling symptoms, she might still have been in a job that gave her so much joy and self-worth or, better still, she might have climbed even higher up the ladder, but her perimenopausal symptoms had wiped out her professional confidence to the point where she felt the only option was to quit. Even medical professionals can miss the symptoms within themselves and plod on.

Priya's story

I'd been a doctor for 20 years and five years ago, when I was a partner in my GP practice, I began to feel that I wasn't up to the job. I've always been punchy at work and pride myself on being at the top of my game, but before I realised I was perimenopausal, I had begun to make small mistakes, such as sending an email with the wrong appointment date. I found myself re-reading emails again and again before clicking 'send'.

I was physically tired – my sleep wasn't what it used to be – and I had mental fatigue. I was also experiencing anxiety for the first time. I initially put it down to my recent bereavement as I'd lost my mother. Even though I'd always suffered badly with PMT, I never thought what was happening could be hormone related. I was a doer, a coper, an achiever – I didn't make excuses. But the penny finally dropped and I tried to discuss it with the other GP partners at my work. Nowadays, we all know where we stand if we were to get pregnant as workplaces have to have a maternity policy, but there is nothing for women at the other side of the reproductive spectrum. I did try to explain perimenopause to them and how it affects women, how it was affecting me – maybe I said it too gently, after all, doctors are no different to patients and it felt embarrassing talking about personal symptoms. I plodded on but working in the NHS is extremely demanding as a GP – you can see 30 patients or more per day. I was exhausted.

Having worked in the NHS for 25 years, I knew I couldn't continue without burning out, losing empathy, making mistakes and losing myself. So, I left. It was an act of self-preservation and I needed to take back control.

I found that exercising in short sharp bursts helped me tackle my anxiety, I'd feel mentally clearer at the end of 20 minutes and found it helped me to sleep better. I looked at my diet – my daughter had turned vegetarian so I decided I would, well almost, and eating a more plant-based diet helped. I felt less bloated, less stodgy, my gut was happier for it. I socialised more and felt happier for it. I also sought out help from my own GP, who I have to say was very understanding. I knew from my history of PMT that hormonal balance was important for me to function and thrive. So, I now am on HRT and have got my motivation and energy back. Also the confidence to set up my own practice independently and I now work as a private GP. I feel I've got me back.

Professional doubt

We think of impostor syndrome as something primarily affecting younger or more junior women – but it can hit hard in perimenopause. Hormonal changes can cause these feelings in perfectly competent, experienced women in their 40s and 50s.

Wondering whether or not you're cut out for your job is a very common part of going through perimenopause. In a recent survey about the impact of menopause on women at work, over half of the respondents said symptoms made their work life worse and a quarter said they had considered leaving their jobs altogether. When you consider that there are 3.5 million women over aged 50 in UK workplaces and a good chunk more aged between 45–50, you can start to see that the numbers affected aren't small fry – even if being perimenopausal at work does feel isolating at times.

Staying in work

Your financial situation might mean you have no choice but to stick with work but, even if you can afford to be more flexible, there are countless benefits that come with staying in your career and continuing to pursue professional opportunities. We're not saying you have to work if you don't want to, but if you do and you feel like you can't because of your hormones, seek help. Remember, your hormones are treatable, but you probably won't get your job back once you've left.

Financial stability and independence

If you contribute to your household finances, your over-all pot would take a hit if you stopped work and if you're the breadwinner or sole earner, giving up work might be an impossible prospect, even if you want to.

Regardless of your situation, maintaining your financial security is a huge reason not to leave work. Even if you don't quit but are considering taking a step back, going part-time, or *not* going for a promotion, think about the impact it'll have on your financial stability. And we're not just talking about your salary, but the knock-on effect on your pension pot, retirement plans, and the loss of other benefits (such as healthcare plans or childcare provisions) that might form part of your package.

Personal identity

Leaving your job – as you know – won't just have an impact on your bank balance. Studies show work gives us purpose and forms an important part of our identities, particu-larly during a time when so much change and transition is happening in our personal lives. If you have children who've left home, you might be suffering with empty nest syndrome at the same time and questioning your work, your value and your sense of purpose at this time. Often now can be the time to re-evaluate and reflect – would carving away at your career be a positive move? Is it time to make a change or to start that project you had been holding back on? Some may call it a midlife crisis; we see it as a midlife re-evaluation.

Of course, we are all more than our job titles, but we underestimate the influence work has on our sense of self at our peril. Beyond this, work gives us status, stimulation and community. Our colleagues form an important part of the circle of people who make up our lives. Your broader network, too, probably enrich your life more than you realise. Taking a career break can make it difficult to keep up with your immediate and extended network. Many women who leave work and attempt to rejoin the same industry later on often find it hard to rebuild these relationships.

Structure and routine

Lastly, our jobs give us a framework from which to plot and plan the rest of our lives. Studies have repeatedly shown the benefits of having a routine for our physical and mental health, and our careers can be an important framework for how we plan our days. If you work, you'll know this already. Our jobs give us structure, motivation and limits, all of which have a positive impact on our overall lives.

The bigger picture

Women over the age of 45 are the fastest-growing demographic in the workplace and – these days – we're expected to work until we're 68. If a woman decides to leave work because of her perimenopausal symptoms, that's 23 years – nearly half of her working life – she's losing out on. But dealing with the pervasiveness of perimenopause isn't just something that affects each woman on an individual level; it's also critical to employers, the economy and society. A report by Oxford Economics suggests that the average cost to replace a lost employee in the UK (as at 2014) was £30k.

Women make brilliant leaders, are great at their jobs, and are assets to their workplaces, so we need to be supported to do our best work, not feel driven out. Plus, every woman lost is a mark against a company's commitment to diversity and inclusion. A woman aged over 45 in the workplace may have already overcome so much: sexual harassment and discrimination, misogynistic bosses and the gender pay gap and, if she's a mother, she will have navigated maternity leave and being a working parent. Losing someone with the resilience it takes to overcome those things should not be underestimated.

The economic impact of often high-earning women leaving their roles around the time of perimenopause is dramatic. Only seven FTSE 100 companies are run by women in a world where women number 50 per cent of the population. Many large companies have quotas that say, for example, by 2030 they want gender parity in their senior leadership team, but unless they support women during perimenopause and address the issues we're talking about in this chapter, they won't get there.

How to cope

Now, it's time for some solutions. Your experience of coping with perimenopause symptoms at work will depend on what kind of job you have. However, whether you're office-based, customer-facing, junior, a manager or a leader, the symptom you're likely to find most difficult is fatigue. When you're suffering from a lack of sleep, you'll feel your energy levels deplete and it'll eventually feel like you're running on an empty tank. If you work in a more physical job – perhaps in retail, a clinical setting, hospitality or service, then this fatigue may well feel physical as well as emotional.

The higher we ascend professionally and the more responsibility we accrue, the harder we might find it when we notice our memory, alertness and focus all taking a hit. This can undermine confidence, and you may find yourself paranoid about doing a simple task, such as sending an email.

The more senior the woman, the more she might think, 'Am I up to this?', and the more those thoughts creep in, the less she'll believe in her abilities. That's when women start to say things like, 'This is a younger woman's job,' even though they might have 25 years' experience behind them and have a wealth of knowledge and talent. Sure, you might need to do some succession planning, but you don't need to opt out. Your symptoms won't last forever, but the impact of leaving a job you love might.

The good news is that there is plenty both you and your employer can do to help make going through the perimenopause while holding down a job easier.

What employers can do

Between the two of us, we've helped businesses like Coutts Bank, Accenture, NatWest Bank and Channel 4, to name a few, to implement menopause policies, so we know there's plenty employers can do to help make work easier for perimenopausal women. Even if your employer doesn't have such a policy (and if that's the case, suggest they develop one), there are lots of measures they could consider implementing:

Reassess uniform policy: if you're getting hot flushes every half an hour and you're wearing clothes that make you feel sticky and uncomfortable, it'll feel suffocating and constrictive, and make the flushes all the more debilitating. Perimenopausal women benefit from uniforms made from breathable fabrics.

Install quiet rooms: find designated rooms or areas where women can go to sit down, breathe through a flush, or calm themselves after a bout of anxiety or panic. Note: this quiet space should also be a cool space!

Water dispensers: having chilled water readily available is something that would benefit many employee groups (like pregnant women, for example), but it's especially helpful for perimenopausal women.

Invest in occupational health: while many businesses and companies offer their staff private medical insurance, it doesn't seem to cover 'menopause' care. Employers should consider specific menopause policies and care as they do for maternity. Examples might be stress management courses, counselling and exercise classes.

Designate menopause champions: yes, we're all menopause champions, but at work, these are people who volunteer their time and act as visible figures that perimenopausal women can talk to about the issues affecting them should they need to.

Be open to flexible working: in some jobs, particularly shift work, flexible working just isn't possible, but in jobs where it is, it can make all the difference to perimenopausal women (well, all women and all men, quite frankly). Whether it's job sharing, compressed hours (working your contracted hours but in fewer days), flexitime (working hours that better suit your schedule, usually with specified 'core hours', e.g. 11am–3pm), working from home, or staggered starting and finishing times, different approaches work for different women, so if you're an employer, make sure you're open to these discussions and, if you're an employee, don't be afraid to ask.

What you can do

Talk about it: if you don't feel ready to have a conversation about your perimenopausal symptoms with your manager, seek out women in a similar situation to you and perhaps set up a network if there's an appetite for it. In a similar way, finding a mentor (whether inside or outside your workplace, but ideally in the same industry) who has been through the perimenopause and can offer you guidance will really help. It's all about actively seeking out ways to feel less isolated in your experience.

Ask for what you need: opening up a dialogue with your employer about the perimenopause can be about as comfortable as having root canal treatment – especially if your manager isn't particularly sensitive to inclusion or hasn't been through it themselves. But your manager will be the person with the power to directly influence your experience and you can't blame your employer for not being attuned to your specific needs unless you vocalise them. Ask specific questions, such as 'Does our company have a menopause policy?', 'What support can HR give me?' 'On a practical note ask, 'Are there desk fans available, and what about a water dispenser?'; 'Can I work flexibly?'

Medication: regardless of your industry, role or seniority, a bespoke prescription of HRT (see page 59) will help to mitigate many of the symptoms women find difficult to cope with at work. You might still be prone to times when you feel more vulnerable and fragile; being on HRT doesn't mean that everything will suddenly smooth out, but it can help you cope better, feel less overwhelmed and minimise anxiety.

Becoming self-employed

We both have experience of running our own businesses while perimenopausal. Between us we have faced a lot of the typical scenarios perimenopausal women experience: looking after elderly parents, teenage kids, relationship breakdowns, grief, divorce and co-parenting. Sometimes these events can throw a spotlight on life as you know it and both of us saw this as a time to reappraise what we wanted from our work. Starting a new business isn't always easy but doing something for you – whatever that is – can be liberating. Also, this time of life is such that you stop pleasing others and don't worry as much about what other people think – you cut out a lot of the crap and just get on with it! It's now or never. What have you got to lose?

What the law says

The law protects women who've suffered from discrimination based on perimenopause. Menopause is covered under three sections of the Equality Act 2010: age, gender and disability discrimination. It's also provided for in the Health and Safety at Work Act 1974. Employers who fail to comply with legislation leave themselves vulnerable to legal action. The first menopause employment tribunal case took place in 2012 and women have since won tribunals based on discrimination pertaining to menopausal symptoms. We know that's not a road many of us want to go down, but you do have that recourse should you need it.

If you feel you've been adversely affected at work due to your symptoms, diarise how your perimenopause has affected your work over two or three months, focusing on two elements: how you think your hormones have affected your performance, and how your workplace reacted and responded to it. It's important to look at both perspectives because, with the benefit of hindsight, we might realise we've been a bit hypersensitive to a situation that turned out to not quite be what we thought it was. Equally though, if you need to take things further, HR or your lawyer will want records.

The future of work

In many ways, we feel optimistic about the future of work, particularly for women. Workplaces are slowly but surely realising they don't need their employees to clock in at 9am and out at 5pm to trust them to do good work. In fact, studies showed that productivity increased during the Covid-19 pandemic. Anything that encourages employers to be more open to flexible working is a good thing for perimenopausal women, but we must tread carefully. The pandemic was also widely reported to have had a detrimental effect on women's career prospects, with them being more vulnerable to losing their jobs, and taking on the lion's share of homeschooling and domestic work. That said, we're hopeful the openness towards flexible working will mean working life improves for perimenopausal women in the long-term.

All the hope in the world, however, won't help if you're at breaking point right now. But think back to Chapter 6, where we discussed mental health and the importance of not making big decisions (like quitting your job or shuttering your business) until you've stabilised your hormones. We'd like to remind you of this and urge you not to throw in the towel at work if you haven't yet done everything you can to improve things. When you feel like resigning on the spot, hold fire: have you worked to balance your hormones? Have you had a conversation with your employer about what they could do to be more understanding and make you more comfortable? Are there any peers you could connect with? Never make a big decision without doing this kind of remedial work first; a hot-headed decision made in a split second could cost you so much security and freedom, and you may later come to regret it.

The bottom line

» You're not alone: perimenopausal symptoms have prompted a quarter of women to consider giving up their jobs.

» Think about what you gain by staying in work: financial security, independence, identity and structure.

» Find coping mechanisms: there's lots your employer can do to help you, and lots you can do to make yourself feel better.

» The law is on your side: don't feel like you are condemned to suffering if you feel you're being discriminated against.

» Have hope: employers are more open to flexible working now than they've ever been; something that will likely make life easier for perimenopausal women.

PART 3
Diet

CHAPTER 10

Nutrition: Nailing The Basics

Life is demanding. The way we eat needn't be.

Food is fundamental to our physical and emotional wellbeing. It powers us through a busy day, helps our brains think straight and staves off illness. Thanks to the immense volume of scientific research linking our nutritional choices to health outcomes, we know that what we eat matters. Yet very few people realise the connection between food and women's health. In this chapter, we'll outline why nourishing your body – not depriving it – is so crucial during perimenopause. We'll introduce you to the seven core nutrition principles for optimal hormone health, show why an anti-inflammatory diet might cut your breast cancer risk by half and explain how the food choices you make each day can help regulate hormone spikes, protect your heart, improve energy, boost mood and reduce cravings.

We'll look at the three main macronutrients – proteins, carbohydrates and fats – that should make up each of your meals and dissect the importance of fibre, which, according to government guidelines, the majority of us need to be doubling. Most importantly, we'll show you while food is crucial to your perimenopause experience, it doesn't have to be complicated. We're all busy and life is demanding. Thankfully, the way we eat needn't be.

Mixed messages

If we were more appreciative of the power of food, we'd be less inclined to let it slip down our priority list. But haywire hormones and busy lives tend to get in the way of eating well. And mixed media messages often muddy the waters, leading us to constantly question. Keto or paleo? Smoothies or juices? Are superfoods still a thing? And what's the deal with fasting?

Positive nutrition

For women already feeling the effects of perimenopause, the simple question of what, when and how to eat can be bewildering, and frequently clients complain they don't have time to sift through the deluge of dietary information they come up against daily. It's true that nutrition has become incredibly complicated and, with the rise of social media, everyone seems to be weighing in not just on what to eat, but all too often, what *not* to eat.

Let's unpack this for a minute. Perimenopause – a time when your body is undergoing significant adjustments – is not a time for deprivation. No good can come from punishing your body into submission because it doesn't look or feel like it used to any more. On the contrary, this is a time for positive nutrition – a time for nourishing yourself, filling up on the good stuff and making small dietary and lifestyle shifts that stack up over time, so they become a way of life.

It's about adding in rather than taking away, balance rather than restriction. Nurturing, yes. Health-giving, definitely. But always with a generous serving of realism.

Facts not fads

The bamboozling nature of perimenopause means it's easy to get sucked into fad diets and influencer hype. The world of nutrition is not black and white. It's a very young science and, as a result, still finding its feet. Ever-emerging research means we're constantly discovering new avenues and re-evaluating previously held theories. It's important to remain open-minded but vigilant about who you take your advice from. Unless they've completed a recognised qualification, health coaches, personal trainers and reality TV stars are *not* reliable sources of up-to-date, evidence-based nutrition information.

Seven core principles for eating optimally during perimenopause

Nutrition is incredibly individual, so what works for one person won't automatically suit someone else. Culture, heritage, background and financial constraints are all factors to be considered. For this reason, try to really tune into *your* body and *your* needs. You don't need to follow any one particular food philosophy and there's absolutely no need for labels. Pick and choose what works for you: we are all unique – from our genes, to our jobs, to our activity levels, to our tastebuds. There are, however, some essential basics that are good practice for pretty much all of us.

1. Balance your blood glucose

Unstable blood glucose is linked to feeling tired, anxious, moody, irritable, lightheaded and forgetful, not to mention gaining weight and craving carbs. Your blood glucose level is the amount of sugar that you have in your blood and, for you to remain healthy, it needs to be kept within certain parameters. When blood-glucose levels peak or trough outside the optimal range, your endocrine (hormone) system is put on high alert and focuses all its attention on trying to stabilise them. This means it has less time for regulating hormones like oestrogen, progesterone and testosterone, potentially resulting in the low libido, PMS-type symptoms, acne, fat around the middle and increased appetite often reported by perimenopausal women.

The rollercoaster effect: your body knows elevated blood-glucose is to be avoided at all costs, so it secretes insulin to remove the circulating glucose from your bloodstream, sending it to your muscles and your liver to be stored for future energy needs. When those two storage tanks are full, insulin sends the glucose to your fat cells. Insulin's sugar clear-up campaign can sometimes be a little over-zealous, which means glucose levels dip below their baseline. It's at this point – usually a couple of hours after eating – that you will experience cravings. It's basically your body's way of trying to urgently replace energy stores.

Highs and lows: the key is to avoid spiking blood glucose too high or allowing it to sink too low. Long-term elevated blood glucose levels increase our risk of obesity, Type 2 diabetes, dementia and heart disease. Low levels make us feel anxious, hangry, shaky and clammy, and can bring on palpitations and headaches. Low levels also cause the body to release cortisol because it sees it as a high stress 'fight-or-flight' situation. But in a horrible twist of biological fate, long-term high levels of cortisol make us more likely to be insulin resistant. So suddenly you're in vicious cycle territory.

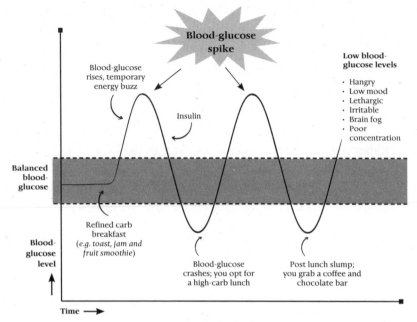

BLOOD-GLUCOSE ROLLERCOASTER

Insulin resistance: insulin resistance occurs when insulin doesn't work as well as it used to. In other words, your body finds it harder to regulate blood-glucose levels. It's important to note there's a sliding scale when it comes to insulin resistance: starting at not processing carbs very efficiently right though to being pre-diabetic. In perimenopausal women insulin resistance can be partly down to lowering oestrogen levels, which help keep a check on insulin, but it can also be down to a diet high in refined carbs, genetics, polycystic ovary syndrome (PCOS), family history, smoking and lack of exercise. Blood glucose levels that swing outside of normal ranges (i.e. spikes and crashes) can drive up inflammation which, if left unchecked, can lead to negative outcomes and increase the risk of viruses and infection.

So, what does all this mean for you and your diet? It doesn't mean you have to avoid carbs completely, but it does mean keeping the following in mind:

» It's hard to get off the blood-sugar rollercoaster once you've jumped on board. So, avoid starting the day with typically high-glucose (sugar) breakfasts such as cereal, orange juice or a croissant and jam. Opt for a protein-based meal like eggs, scrambled tofu or Greek yoghurt instead.

» Be aware that refined carbs can spike blood-sugar levels quite dramatically. We're talking white bread, white pasta, pies, breakfast cereals, muffins and pancakes.

» Movement after a meal can help bring down high glucose levels. So, if you've enjoyed a delicious bowl of pasta and some dessert, try going for a walk afterwards.

» Choose complex carbs that are released slowly: wholegrains like brown rice or jumbo oats, beans, vegetables and berries.

» It's not just food that has an impact: caffeine, nicotine and alcohol (especially on an empty stomach) can also trigger blood-glucose spikes.

» If you want to eat something sweet, such as a biscuit or a slice of cake, tagging it on to the end of a meal, as opposed to eating it as a snack, will reduce the spike.

» Have a craving for something sweet? Wait 20 minutes to see if it dissipates. Quite often it will as your blood-glucose levels will have stabilised and the craving will pass.

» Add protein and/or fibre to carb-based meals and snacks to counteract sugar spikes.

» Eat fruit whole rather than juicing it ... even better, add in a few nuts: have some pumpkin-seed butter with your banana; add an egg to your avocado toast.

» We don't all respond to glucose in foods the same way. You can find out how you react by wearing a continuous glucose monitor that measures your response and gives you feedback via an app (see page 272).

» Stress and sleep both impact blood-glucose levels. See Chapter 8 for useful sleep tips.

» The more muscle you have, the better your insulin sensitivity is, even at rest. We look at resistance training in closer detail in Chapter 13.

» Intermittent fasting (IF) (see page 270) has been shown to help with insulin resistance in some cases.

» Increased weight around the middle, which gives you more of an 'apple shape', is a sign you may be more resistant to insulin. Get your tape measure out – according to the NHS, your waist should ideally be less than 80cm.

» Signs of insulin resistance include fatigue, high triglycerides, high cholesterol, skin tags and acanthosis nigricans: dark patches of skin on the neck, armpits and sometimes groin. If you think you might be at risk, ask your doctor to test your glucose tolerance and/or your fasting insulin.

2. Eat like a Mediterranean

While there's no such a thing as a perimenopause diet, the traditional Mediterranean way of eating is a good bench-mark to guide you on your eating journey. Why? Essentially because it has potent anti-inflammatory properties, contains little to no processed foods, is low in sugar and high in fibre. These factors make sense at any time of life, but are particularly valid during perimenopause when the body is under so much stress. Where there's stress, inflammation usually follows and it is widely accepted that inflammation is the precursor to many of the chronic diseases and auto-immune conditions that women are susceptible to, including arthritis, Alzheimer's, heart disease and hypothyroidism.

So what does the Mediterranean diet look like in real terms? As you'd expect, there is a strong focus on vegetables, fruit, legumes (lentils, chickpeas, peas and beans), grains, olive oil, nuts and seeds, herbs and spices, alongside some fish and seafood, moderate dairy and a limited amount of meat. Bear in mind the diet is a guide rather than written in stone and can be adjusted according to your taste, budget and preferences (see box).

Coronary heart disease kills twice as many women in the UK as breast cancer. Because oestrogen is cardio-protective, low levels increase your risk of a cardiovascular related event significantly, something to be aware of as you transition into perimenopause and through to later life. Numerous studies link the Mediterranean diet with a lower risk of heart disease, strokes, depression, Type 2 diabetes, obesity, dementia and some cancers. In fact, the Lyon Diet Heart Study found that a group of participants who followed the Mediterranean diet were 45 per cent less likely to die over the four-year duration of the programme compared to their counterparts who were following a low-fat diet. Interestingly, the Mediterranean diet isn't just about what you eat, but how you eat too. Mediterraneans tend to spend longer eating their meals and enjoy them as part of a wider community, with friends and family. Worth thinking about when you're next bolting down a sandwich hunched over your laptop.

The Mediterranean diet

Make the Mediterranean diet work for you:

» Tinned beans, lentils and chickpeas are budget-friendly and save time. Try ready-cooked pouches for ease.

» Olive oil comes in a huge range of prices, so buy what you can afford. Recent studies have shown extra virgin olive oil (EVOO) has a smoke point of around 210 degrees centigrade, which is perfectly suited to most types of cooking. To be more budget friendly though, you could cook with olive oil and save your best EVOO for dressings and dips.

» Grow your own mini herb garden on your windowsill.

» Bulk-buy dry goods like grains, nuts and seeds to get the best value. Store in reusable airtight containers.

» It's never too late to start. In a study of over 10,000 women, those who embarked on a Mediterranean way of eating during midlife were more likely to live past 70 than those who followed a Western-style diet.

3. Get more plants on your plate

It is widely accepted that a plant-focused diet (it doesn't have to be solely vegan) is beneficial for all aspects of health and this chimes with the Mediterranean way of eating as described above. Not only do plant-based foods contain fibre, they're also a brilliant source of vitamins, minerals, antioxidants and phytonutrients. As a bonus they're filling, accessible and can be relatively inexpensive if you opt for UK-grown produce.

A healthy eating plan that includes plenty of colourful fruits and vegetables can help lower your risk of chronic diseases such as heart disease, obesity, high blood pressure, diabetes and some cancers – all of which we become more susceptible to as the protective effects of our hormones decline. But perhaps the most advantageous aspect of eating plant-based foods is that they provide essential food, called prebiotics, that help your gut microbes thrive (see Chapter 12). Good gut health is vital to you at this time of life, affecting everything from your hormones to your mood to your immunity.

A good way to ensure you're getting as much diversity as possible is to 'eat the rainbow'; this sounds trite but is actually a nice visual reminder to keep your meals colourful, fresh and varied. If you've got kids, get them involved with buying, prepping and cooking. Encourage younger children to make a chart where they tick off the different colours of foods they eat in a week – hummus, dips, fruit purees on porridge, smoothies, mini veg muffins and pesto sauces are easy ways to diversify their diet, and yours.

According to research from Imperial College London, eating eight portions (a portion = approximately three heaped tablespoons) of vegetables and two of fruit a day could prevent almost 8 million premature deaths a year, but don't get too hung up on the numbers; think of this as a guide rather than the law and even if you only manage ten portions once or twice a week that's still worth shouting about. If you're nowhere near, don't fret. Take a look at your current diet and track how many fruit and vegetables you eat daily, then try to increase by a portion or two every week.

Organic produce and farmers' markets are all well and good, but they're not always affordable and they certainly aren't essential. Frozen fruit and vegetables bought from your local supermarket will keep for a few months, is affordable, just as nutritious as fresh (sometimes more) and often mean less food waste. Frozen produce has the added advantage of being 'snap frozen' at source, which locks in nutrients, compared to supposedly fresh options, which spend time in transit only to sit on supermarket shelves or wait in your fridge for days. In a study carried out by the University of California, vitamin C was found to be higher in frozen corn, green beans and blueberries than in their fresh counterparts.

Five easy ways to eat more fruit and veg for less.

1. Pre-packaged supermarket produce is often more expensive than buying the items loose – i.e. five bananas sold in a bag vs. five individual bananas. Avoiding means you save on plastic too.
2. Try adding frozen greens, carrots, sweetcorn and peas to soups, curries and stews. Frozen spinach and courgette works really well in fruit smoothies and usually can't be detected, even by discerning little ones.
3. Beans, lentils and chickpeas count as one of your fruit and veg intake (that includes spaghetti hoops and baked beans too, though try to go for the low-sugar versions).
4. Pad out pasta dishes, casseroles, bolognese sauces and lasagnes with lentils and beans.
5. Bulk-buy at a grocers rather than a supermarket as it tends to be cheaper. Opting for what's in season can halve the cost. Consider splitting the bill and the spoils with a friend or family member. Wash, chop and freeze anything that doesn't look like it'll get used in time.

4. Power up on protein

We can't stress enough the importance of protein – even if you do nothing else, make this the star of the show when it comes to planning your meals. It provides the literal building blocks for every cell in your body – from hormones, bones and DNA to skin, nails and hair. Without it, we can't function. We need it for energy production, sleep, mood and libido; it's also great for curbing cravings, filling you up and keeping on top of hunger. In a nutshell, protein ticks a lot of boxes when it comes to perimeno-pause symptoms.

Sometime around our mid-30s, we start to experience muscle loss (known as sarcopenia), which becomes more pronounced around perimenopause thanks to the loss of oestrogen, progesterone and testosterone, and continues to decline in our 50s, 60s and beyond. Muscle mass is some-thing we want to hang on to at all costs: for strength, yes, but also because muscle ramps up your metabolism and helps with weight management (see page 238).

One study found women consuming high amounts of protein per day (around 90g) had a 30 per cent lower risk of muscle loss. If you haven't already cottoned on, protein is a veritable powerhouse and the key to better ageing.

The current recommended intake of protein is 0.75g per kilogram of body weight per day, but this is conservative. Perimenopausal women should be looking at around 1.2g of protein per kilogram of body weight per day (a little more if you're very active, work out a lot, have recently been ill or have a physically demanding job). So a 70kg woman needs around 70–100g of protein a day, ideally split across meals as your body can't break down large amounts in one go. If weighing food isn't your thing, an easy way to gauge quan-tities is to think of a portion the size of your palm at every meal: a chicken breast, half a cup of lentils, three eggs or half a block of tofu.

Protein intake

Here's an example of a 70kg woman's ideal protein intake for one day:

Breakfast: two eggs and a mackerel fillet with toast

Lunch: soup with half a can of green lentils added

Dinner: chicken breast with brown rice and steamed edamame beans

Snack: small pot Greek yoghurt with raspberries and a tablespoon of mixed seeds

---

High-quality proteins are 'complete' i.e. they contain all nine essential amino acids and are found in animal products and one or two plant-based sources (see below). This means if you're vegan or vegetarian, you need to eat a range of plant-based sources to ensure you're getting the full amino acid profile. This is relatively easy if you're consuming plenty of legumes such as lentils, peas, chickpeas and beans. Even if you're a meat eater, it's worth trying to up your plant protein intake for the variety and fibre they provide.

Complete protein sources: meat, fish, dairy, eggs, quinoa, soya, buckwheat, seitan, tempeh, tofu, edamame beans, amaranth, nutritional yeast.

Almost complete: hemp and chia (both quite low in lysine).

Incomplete plant-based proteins: beans, lentils, chickpeas, nuts, nut butters, seeds, brown/black/wild rice, rye, wheat, spelt, oats, teff and barley.

Complete protein combinations: rice and beans with your veggie stew; sunflower seeds sprinkled on lentil soup; peanut butter and wholewheat crackers.

Protein powders

Protein powders can be convenient if you're on the move or pushed for time, but they're often expensive and don't come with all the other nutrients, minerals and vitamins a proper meal would provide. There are lots on the market of varying quality, taste and cost and there are many vegan options (usually made from a pea and bean or rice blend) if you want to avoid whey. Try a sample first before investing. Lots of health-food shops stock single sachets so you can see if you like the taste and texture before you buy a larger quantity.

Some people find protein powder upsets their stomach, especially if it is consumed too close to the end of a workout. This is because your body is still in flight-or-flight mode and not in the mood for digesting. We used to think there was a 30-minute window post-workout when muscle synthesis was optimal; now we know that as long as you have some protein within a couple of hours you'll be fine. And if for some reason you don't, it's certainly not the end of the world. Many shakes and supplements also have artificial sweeteners and sugar alcohols (look for mannitol, xylitol, sorbitol … anything ending in -ol on the ingredients list), which can cause cramping and bloating. Always check the labels before you buy.

5. Don't fear fats

Forget the scaremongering of previous times – fats are back in favour. The fact is we need some fats in our diet, especially during perimenopause. Our sex hormones – oestrogen, progesterone and testosterone – are made from the choles-terol found in saturated fats. Our brains are no less than 60 per cent fat. Fats also makes up our cell membrane walls, including the myelin sheath that surrounds brain neurons, and they're needed for us to absorb vitamins A, D, E and K. A balanced meal should always include some healthy fat: a quarter of an avocado, a matchbox-sized amount of nuts and seeds or a tablespoon of olive oil. The rub is that some people have taken this to extremes and are now advising cooking everything in coconut oil and adding butter to your morning caffeine hit: aka bulletproof coffee.

But what about the link between saturated fat and heart disease? Good question, and one of the most divisive topics in nutrition science today. What we do know is that some studies show saturated fats aren't implicated in heart disease to such a degree as they used to be, but they're still not a health food. As with everything, it comes down to balance and quality. Get the majority of your fats from unsaturated sources such as oily fish, olive oil, avocados, nuts and seeds, and include moderate amounts of saturated fats like butter, red meat and coconut oil. As a rule, we tend to eat far more Omega 6 sources of fats (highly processed seeds and vege-table oils like sunflower and soybean oil) than Omega 3. Omega 3 fats have anti-inflammatory properties, whereas Omega 6 fats – in large amounts – appear to have a poten-tially pro-inflammatory effect. The best Omega 3 source is oily fish (see below). If you're not eating the recommended amount (twice a week), it's wise to supplement.

One thing everyone agrees on is that trans fats are damaging to heart health. Most manufacturers have agreed to stop using them in the UK, but they can still be found in some foods like margarine and doughnuts. Look for 'hydrogenated oil' or 'mono and diglycerides of fatty acids' on labels and avoid where possible.

Saturated fats: butter, coconut oil, coconut cream, lard, ghee, palm oil, red meat, cheese.

Unsaturated fats: avocado, olives, oils (flax, olive, rapeseed, sesame seed), oily fish (anchovies, herring, mackerel, pilchards, salmon, sardines, trout, whitebait), nuts, seeds.

6. Stop cancelling carbs

Headaches, irritability, fatigue, constipation, sugar cravings, high cholesterol and bloating can all be down to a lack of complex carbs in your diet. Yet despite the fact these common perimenopause symptoms could potentially be improved so easily, carbs are still plagued by controversy and often shunned by women. Many just can't seem to get past the widely held view that carbs make you inflamed, sluggish and unable to lose fat. This isn't true. Carbs contain just 4 calories per gram (compared to fats, which clock in at 9 calories per gram), they fuel our muscles, pack in fibre and, when chosen wisely, are an excellent source of vitamins and minerals. Your brain is the hungriest organ in your body, using up around 20 per cent of the energy you consume in a day in its resting state, and carbs are its favourite food. Research suggests our brains use the equivalent of over 400 calories of glucose a day, which goes some way to explaining why low-carb diets can blunt your mental acuity, make your mood swing wildly and give you brain fog.

The issue is that 'carbs' all get lumped together, but there are good-quality, complex carbs that it makes sense to include in your diet in reasonable portions. The other type – the more refined variety – are definitely worth moderating. Complex carbs (mostly derived from plants) provide sustained energy that's released slowly over time. As we hit perimenopause, we become slightly less insulin – and therefore carb – sensitive (see page 162), so it's wise to avoid high amounts of refined, simple carbs (mostly from processed foods) as these are more likely to spike your blood sugars and launch you on to the much-maligned insulin response rollercoaster (see page 161). So far so good: fewer biscuits, cakes, croissants, muffins and refined grain/white flour products is not exactly rocket science when it comes to healthy eating messages. But what about potatoes, pasta and bread? These are known as starchy carbs and they often get a bad rap, especially when it comes to weight gain. They are in no way inherently 'bad' for you, but when paired with calorie-rich sauces or when deep fried, they're easy to overeat. No one wolfs down bowlfuls of plain pasta, but add in some creamy carbonara sauce and a generous layer of parmesan and things start to take a different slant. It pays to stay mindful – these starchy carbs are pretty energy-dense foods and some days you might simply need more of them than others. Be aware of how active you are – if you're sitting at a desk all day, you won't need as many high-starch carbs as a cleaner or builder might.

In the table below there are some suggestions to replace simple carbs that spike blood-sugar levels with those that allow a slower release of glucose.

Simple carbs	Easy swaps
Bagels, crackers, white bread	Wholegrain wraps
Instant oats	Steel cut/jumbo oats

Simple carbs	Easy swaps
Rice cakes	Dark rye crackers
White rice and white pasta	Al dente* wholewheat pasta
Cereal	Homemade granola
Fruit juice	Eat the whole fruit
* not over-cooking pasta helps slow the release of glucose into the blood.	

One of the biggest arguments for not following a very low-carb diet, such as the keto diet, is that you're missing out on valuable sources of fibre, which affects your gut microbiota and can leave you constipated. As well as making you feel bloated, constipation can cause you to strain on the toilet, which impacts your pelvic floor.

7. Make friends with fibre

Many of the most common complaints in clinic – bloating, constipation, weight gain, even symptoms like tender breasts caused from oestrogen dominance when levels are fluctuating – can be helped by increasing dietary fibre. The benefits of all types of fibre-filled foods (most commonly found in vegetables, fruit, beans, peas and chickpeas) are well documented – from lowering cholesterol and avoiding constipation to slowing the release of glucose into our blood and helping us feel full. Yet we're still not getting enough.

The current recommendation is a fibre intake of 30g a day; most of us get only just over half that. Soluble fibre in the form of oats and fruit, such as figs and pears, helps maintain healthy cholesterol levels and feed our good gut bacteria (see page 221). Insoluble fibre from things like wholegrains (see list below), nuts and seeds is useful for bulking up poo and making it easier to push out. A quick word on wholegrains which, thanks to the paleo diet, seem to be getting a bad rap lately, with lots of people cutting them from their diets. The association with inflammation is largely unfounded. In fact, in one large study, overweight adults who changed from a refined to an unrefined wholegrain diet actually lost weight and reduced inflammation. Wholegrains are a rich source of B vitamins, magnesium, iron, selenium and phosphorus, and numerous controlled trials link them to a reduced risk of developing diabetes, heart disease, Type 2 diabetes, weight gain and even some cancers.

Your dietary choices are yours and you know how you react to individual foods better than anybody else, but if you omit entire food groups ensure that you're replacing the lost nutrients from elsewhere in your diet. Speak to a nutritionist for specific guidance.

Eating more grains

Some ideas to get more diversity into your diet:

Wholegrains: brown/black/wild rice, rye, wheat, spelt, oats, teff and barley.

Pseudo grains: not technically grains but prepared and eaten in the same way – quinoa, freekah, amaranth, buckwheat, millet.

A good way to see if a supposedly wholegrain shopping item, let's say bread, is high in fibre is to check the label and multiply the grams of fibre by ten. If the number you get is bigger than the grams of total carbohydrate, you're on to a winner. Add fibre into your diet gradually, as sudden increases can cause digestive issues like bloating and wind.

The table below shows the approximate amount of fibre in foods.

Food	Fibre content
1 cupped hand of green peas (boiled, 100g)	4.5g
One-third of a can of chickpeas (75g)	5g
Wholemeal bread (2 slices)	5g
1 pear (medium)	5.5g
1 apple (medium)	4.5g
Small baked potato (180g)	5g
2 cupped handfuls of wholewheat pasta (cooked, 150g)	5g
Ground flaxseed (1tbsp)	3.5g
Lentils (100g)	8g
(Adapted from: bda.uk.com)	

A 30g-day of fibre might look something like this:

Breakfast
Small bowl of porridge made from oats = 5g
1 fresh fig = 2g
20 raspberries = 2g

Lunch
1 medium baked sweet potato = 6g
A cupped hand of roasted chickpeas = 8g

Dinner
Bowl of red lentil dahl with cupped hand of mixed veg = 7g

Total: 30g

12 easy ways to increase fibre in your diet

1. Keep the skin on fruit and vegetables where possible. Tip: roasting a whole butternut squash softens the skin, tastes great and saves a massive amount of time and effort.
2. Add 2 tablespoons of ground flaxseed to your meals and snacks throughout the day – for example, to smoothies, porridge, salads and yoghurt.
3. Add lentils, beans, peas and chickpeas to soups, stews, curries and sauces. Tip: buy ready-cooked pouches for convenience.
4. Choose wholemeal pasta and wholegrain bread.
5. Add nuts and seeds to your breakfast. They taste great with yoghurt, porridge, chia pudding, and even eggs.
6. Try sprinkling psyllium husks over yoghurt or add to soups, granola or overnight oats. Start with 1 teaspoon and work up slowly; if tolerated well (i.e. there is no digestive discomfort or excessive bowel movements), go up to 3 tablespoons a day.
7. Overnight oats are a brilliant and quick breakfast and a useful source of insoluble fibre. Combine 45g oats with 100ml milk of your choice, 3 tablespoons of yoghurt and 1 tablespoon of chia seeds in a jar with a lid. Mix well and leave overnight in the fridge. Add toppings and sweeten, as desired, in the morning.
8. Avoid long-term low-carb diets. Carbs = fibre. Just make sure you opt for good-quality, complex carbs (see page 173).

9. Replace crisps with popcorn for a high-fibre snack.
10. Fibre-dense fruits include pears, figs, kiwi fruit, raspberries, blackberries and apples.
11. Check labels: high-fibre food is considered to have 6g (or more) fibre per 100g.
12. Like oats in the morning? Rotate them with other high-fibre grains: rye, spelt, buckwheat and quinoa flakes are good options.

The bottom line

» Positive nutrition is the way forward. Perimenopause is hard enough, so be kind to yourself by giving your body the goodness it needs, not depriving it through restrictive diets.

» Eat more plants: ensuring around half your plate is made up from vegetables, salad greens, beans and pulses is one thing pretty much every nutrition professional agrees on.

» Pack in the protein: eat a palm-sized portion at each meal.

» Choose wholefoods vs processed, where possible: nature packages foods in such a way that they contain the extra nutrients and enzymes needed to aid absorption.

» Be a savvy shopper: cans, tins, pouches and frozen food can be game changers in the kitchen.

» Try to keep your blood-glucose levels nice and steady by starting the day with a protein-based breakfast.

» Fat stats: unsaturated fats are in, trans fat are out and saturated fats are ok in moderation.
» You don't need to label your diet: flexible eating means you respond to your body's changing needs.
» Fill up on fibre: it's linked to better overall health and reduces the risk of more than 70 chronic diseases, including heart disease, Type 2 diabetes and several cancers. Just remember to go low and slow when increasing fibre as your gut needs time to adjust. And make sure you hydrate well.

CHAPTER 11

Eat to Beat Your Symptoms

Increase your appetite for feeling good.

In the previous chapter, you learnt the importance of balancing your blood-sugar levels and got to grips with the fundamentals of a balanced diet. You may not necessarily be nailing eight portions of vegetables and two portions of fruit a day (these things take time), but hopefully you have a clearer idea of the direction you'd like your diet to be going in. In this chapter, we are going to take a closer look at what it means to eat for perimenopause and how to increase your appetite for feeling good. We'll look at the most prevalent symptoms and how what you consume – or in some cases don't consume – can help or hinder. Not all will apply to you (hopefully!), so feel free to skim your way through to the most relevant sections. Bear in mind, many of these conditions are rather complex, not to mention nuanced, so the information is for general guidance and not intended to replace a detailed nutrition or medical consultation.

Anxiety and mood swings

There's a strong association between food and mood: our state of mind can shape the food choices we make, and certain foods can impact how we feel. Low mood can lead to erratic eating behaviours, including skipping meals, bingeing or comfort eating. This can impact your overall nutrient intake and lead to blood-sugar imbalances that cause anxiety and mood swings. One of the most important things you can do for anxiety is to balance your blood sugar (see page 160) because when levels drop, your body releases the stress hormones cortisol and adrenaline. Stress disrupts progesterone, aka your 'grounding' hormone, which then has a knock-on effect with mood, irritability, sleep and feeling calm.

Here are three ways food can help your mood:

1. Start with the 'Key 3'
The easiest way to stabilise blood sugar – and ensure your mood stays on an even keel – is to check your plate contains the Key 3: protein, fibre and fats. Having all three elements in meals will help you feel satiated, keep cravings at bay later in the day and remove the need for snacking.

2. Unshackle from sugar
Sugar makes you feel high, but what goes up must come down. And when you do come off your sugar buzz, you're invariably left feeling irritable, snappy and shattered. Let's not be puritanical about this, though – there's a time and place to enjoy sugar, but ideally we want it to be periodic rather than daily. High-sugar foods don't fill you up, they tend to be low in nutrients and they're not always great

for your gut health. Here are a few ways to reduce your sugar load:

» Try a teaspoon of vanilla bean paste in your porridge or Greek yoghurt. It has a rich flavour, but doesn't contain added sugar.

» Fill your fruit bowl and think of it as your first port of call for snacks (ideally eaten with a few nuts to stabilise your body's blood-sugar response).

» Swap your milk/white chocolate for dark chocolate. If you're new to dark chocolate, start with 40 per cent cocoa and work your way up to 85, 90 or even 100 per cent. The darker the chocolate, the less added sugar it contains (it's also a source of iron and antioxidants).

» Swap sweetened yoghurt (often labelled 'low fat') for authentic Greek yoghurt (not to be confused with 'Greek style', which has much less protein). If you're vegan, opt for unsweetened soya yoghurt. You can always add a little honey, vanilla bean paste or maple syrup, but at least you're in control of how much – use a spoon to gauge; don't pour from the pot.

» Stewed apples or pears provide natural sweetness, as well as fibre.

» Enhance foods with spices instead of sugar; try ginger, allspice, cinnamon or nutmeg. These taste great, boast numerous healthy plant chemicals (for more on polyphenols, see page 227) and can be used liberally. Small studies link cinnamon with reduced sugar cravings and research is currently looking into certain spices having potential anti-Alzheimer's properties.

» A Medjool date stuffed with a teaspoon of nut butter is a delicious, high-fibre snack that hits the sweet spot.

Eat straight from the freezer for a lovely, caramel-like texture.

» Agave, coconut sugar, honey and date syrup are still types of sugar and your body treats them pretty much the same as it does white table sugar. Enjoy them, but don't think they're any 'better' or 'healthier' than the white stuff.

» Inulin (made from chicory root) is a useful sugar swap as it's high in fibre (it's a prebiotic), but has a natural sweet taste. You can buy it in big bags from most heath-food shops and online. Add a teaspoon to porridge, use it in baking or add to tea and coffee.

3. Magnificent magnesium

We've mentioned the importance of magnesium and sleep (see page 139), but it also supports the nervous system so a deficiency can leave you feeling anxious and fatigued. High-stress states (hello perimenopause!) can deplete magnesium stores dramatically, so it's worth taking a good hard look at where you're getting your intake. Good sources include dark green leafy vegetables (chard, chicory, kale, spinach, rocket, watercress, romaine lettuce), nuts and seeds. See page 253 for advice on magnesium supplementation.

Other food and mood factors

» Caffeine makes many people feel jittery and anxious. Replace it with herbal or green tea, which contains caffeine but also L-theanine, which calms the nervous system.

» Simple carbs (refined sugars) (see page 174) send your blood glucose into disarray and disrupt neurotransmitter function, which can exacerbate feelings of anxiety.

» Get plenty of vitamin C and all the B vitamins, as they are needed to support adrenal health, but are depleted fairly dramatically by stress (see page 248).

» Iron and B vitamins support the nervous system. Low levels of B3, B6 and B12 are linked to irritability, low mood and depression. See page 193 for information on iron and to ensure you're getting all your B vitamins. It might be worth considering taking a B complex supplement (see page 255).

» CBD oil (see page 261) is being marketed as the new anxiety-busting kid on the block.

» Sleep and exercise both have a marked impact on anxiety levels. Reducing stress is easier said than done – and for most of us it's a work in progress, but for approaches that might help, go to page 248 and see Chapter 8 for sleep strategy reminders.

» The lauded SMILES trial showed that eating a Mediterranean-style diet (see page 166) for 12 weeks (alongside therapeutic interventions) helped to reduce anxiety. Yet another thumbs up for this way of eating.

» Ask your doctor to test your vitamin D levels to check if you need to supplement (see page 256).

Bladder problems

Women commonly experience bladder conditions during perimenopause, but often just put up with them because they think it's simply part of getting older. It might be common but it's not normal, so please don't suffer in silence. There are lots of ways to turn symptoms around.

Urinary leakage

We have oestrogen receptors all over our bodies, including our pelvic floor. Oestrogen is needed for strength, collagen production and elasticity in the ligaments that hold the pelvic floor muscles in place. This is why many women find they start to suffer from stress (when coughing or jumping) and urge (unable to hold in their urine) incontinence as they head into perimenopause. There's a wealth of information online regarding the best way to strengthen your pelvic floor (we recommend the NHS's Squeezy app for information and for reminders). In terms of diet, there are also additions and omissions you can make to reduce your chances of leaking:

» Limit alcohol and caffeine as they encourage your kidneys to produce more urine.
» Drink plenty of water. This sounds counterintuitive, but if you're not drinking enough water, your wee gets more concentrated, which can irritate your bladder.
» Avoid getting constipated as bearing down can really exacerbate pelvic floor issues (see below and go to page 178 for ways to add fibre to your diet).
» Spicy food, citrus fruits and fizzy drinks can all cause the bladder to spasm, which increases urge and frequency.

UTIs (urinary tract infections)
For medical guidance, see page 28. From a dietary point of view, consider:

» Reducing caffeine and alcohol intake as both can irritate the bladder lining.
» Drinking plenty of water as it dilutes urine, helping to prevent and cure UTIs.
» D-Mannose is a supplement that has been shown to help prevent the bad bacteria sticking to the walls of the bladder. The dosages that have been used in studies

for prevention are 2g a day, and for an active episode 1g three times a day (so 3g in total) for 14 days.

» Some women find a 'women's health' probiotic aimed specifically at colonising the vaginal microbiome helps prevent further UTIs.

Brain changes

The brain consumes around 20 per cent of the food we eat every day (see page 173). It's by far your body's hungriest organ, so it stands to reason you need to feed it effectively. It requires energy from calories to function well (hence the reason you may not fire on all cylinders when you go on a restrictive diet), but also plenty of nutrients to fuel the production of 'happy' signallers, such as dopamine and serotonin.

Omega 3 and brain function

Omega 3 is a type of long-chain fatty acid and an essential component of every cell in the body, particularly when it comes to our brain and eyes. It's deemed 'essential' as we can't make it, so we have to get it from our diet or from supplements. The two most important compounds in Omega 3s are called DHA and EPA and many studies link them to improved mental health.

Brain boosters

To get your weekly dose of Omega 3, aim for two servings of oily fish a week (tinned, fresh or frozen) (see page 172). If you don't like the taste of fish, you can supplement with fish oil. If you're vegetarian or vegan, go for an algae-based supplement.

There are lots of fish oils and algae supplements on the market (see page 254).

While it's true that nuts and seeds contain Omega 3, it's the inactive form called ALA, which your body has to convert into the active forms, DHA and EPA. This conversion is extremely inefficient, so while foods like walnuts, chia seeds, flaxseed and hemp are good sources of vitamin E and fibre, they're not actually great sources of brain-friendly Omega 3.

Fogginess

Your brain mass is about three-quarters water. When that level dips, even a little, it can result in sluggishness, fatigue, brain fog, sleep problems and low mood. If you're one of those people who switches off when you're told to drink water, it's time to have a re-think. Staying hydrated can really help with focus and mental performance. Drink a glass of water when you wake up and have a refillable bottle on your desk or in your bag to remind you to keep topping up. Make it more interesting with mint, rosemary, cucumber, slices of fresh ginger and lemon or lime. Sipping frequently, rather than chugging back huge amounts in one go, will help curb the need for frequent toilet dashes.

Digestive health

Fluctuating hormone levels can have a marked effect on digestive health. Similarly to in early pregnancy, changes in the levels of follicle stimulating hormone (FSH) can lead to feelings of nausea. Oestrogen helps with peristalsis – the movement of food through the digestive tract – so when levels dwindle it stands to reason that gut issues like a gurgling tummy, wind and burping might follow.

Bloating

Some bloating after a meal is completely normal, but if it's frequent, uncomfortable or affects your quality of life then it needs to be investigated further. As a general guide, if you wake up bloated, it's important to rule out potential gynaecological issues. Digestive-related bloating, on the other hand, tends to build up throughout the day and is usually relieved by a bowel movement. Most women immediately think of culprits like dairy or gluten and start eliminating these from their diet, which is often unnecessary. There are lots of different reasons you might experience bloating (see below), but the main trigger is a silent one: stress. When you're stressed, you produce less stomach acid and digestive enzymes, which means an increased risk of bloating and gas. Stress also diverts blood flow away from the gut, which makes digestion – and nutrient absorption – even less efficient. So, before you embark on a hugely restrictive diet, consider keeping a rudimentary symptom diary to try to work out your trigger(s). Factors to think about logging, aside from stress, might include poor sleep, foods like garlic and onions, high-histamine foods (see page 208) and caffeine. Tracking helps to highlight any unexpected patterns.

Other factors that can trigger bloating:

» An increase in gas-producing foods, like broccoli, beans and cauliflower.
» Eating in front of something like a laptop or TV. Studies have found we consume more – and eat quicker – when we eat alongside distractions.

» Eating too fast.
» Poor posture: when you're slouched, your digestive system can't work optimally. This can lead to bloating, burping, reflux and trapped wind.
» Food intolerances. These are much less common than people think, but if you suspect one, speak to your doctor. A registered nutritionist or dietitian can support you through an elimination and re-introduction diet.
» Alcohol can cause bloating because it irritates the lining of the stomach and reduces the amount of digestive enzymes you produce.
» Long-term bloating can be due to more serious illnesses, so if your symptoms are continuous or accompanied by vomiting, nausea, changes in bowel habit or weight loss, speak to a doctor.
» With the exception of lactose intolerance, which can be diagnosed via a breath test, you cannot diagnose food intolerances through testing, so please don't waste your money on expensive kits.

To help with bloating:

» Try taking 1–2 peppermint oil capsules (like Colpermin) 30 minutes before meals.
» Chew your food thoroughly – around 20 bites per mouthful.
» Avoid sitting in tight clothing for long periods: belts, active wear and high-waisted jeans can all be problematic.
» Try eating smaller meals spread throughout the day.
» Some protein powders can make people bloated and gassy, especially if consumed too fast. Take your time.

» Fizzy drinks, smoking and chewing gum can cause you to swallow air.

» If you eat lots of salt, try cutting back. Guidelines recommend no more than a teaspoon a day, but it's often hidden in processed foods.

» Try abdominal massage to release trapped gas. See diagram below.

» Look out for sugar alcohols (polyols) on ingredients labels – these usually end in 'ol', such as maltitol, xylitol, erythritol and sorbitol.

» Have you upped your fibre recently? You might need to rein it in until your symptoms subside then increase again, but slowly.

» Go for a walk. Movement can really help to get things moving.

» Peppermint, fennel or ginger tea can be soothing. Make your own ginger tea by chopping fresh ginger and putting it in a saucepan of gently simmering water for 30 minutes. Strain before drinking (and try adding a squeeze of lemon).

» Take a few deep breaths before each meal (try the 3–4–5 method on page 134) to ensure you're in rest-and-digest mode.

» Digestive enzymes can help in some cases. Take before a meal (after can work too if you forget).

» A hot-water bottle can help to relax gut muscles.

» Who hasn't farted in a yoga class? Try the wind-relieving pose Pawanmuktasana to bring one on.

» Some women find eating bitter foods before a meal helps as they encourage bile production, which aids digestion. For example, try some rocket with olive oil and a squeeze of lemon.

Constipation

You may find you're much less frequent, or your stools are harder to push out, when you hit perimenopause. Once again, there are a lot of reasons: from being more sedentary to losing the 'propelling' effects that oestrogen has on gut motility. Dehydration – lack of water or increased alcohol – can also be a cause, but the most common is – yep, you guessed it – stress. Most of us should naturally experience a surge of the stress hormone, cortisol, first thing in the morning. This is normal and actually helpful as it's the signal for us to wake up. For many people it also works to trigger a bowel movement. But if you're chronically stressed – i.e. feeling the effects over a long period of time – your body may well put bowel movements on hold while it deals with what it sees as more important bodily functions. In the past these would have been running away from a bear that wanted to eat you, but these days it's more likely to be dealing with a full inbox or trying to get to work on time. Other factors that can slow things down include long-distance travel, unfamiliar toilets (we've all been there) and thyroid issues. This last one requires a trip to your doctor and getting some tests done, but before we go there, let's ensure we're getting the basics right:

» Are you drinking enough fluid? We need on average two litres per day and the bowels use a lot of this, so upping your water consumption can make things a little easier. We also need water to enable fibre to do its job properly, which leads nicely on to the next point.

» Are you cutting carbs? They provide fibre, but also help us produce serotonin, which is needed to help with peristalsis: the movement of food through the digestive system. Not enough might mean a sluggish, 'depressed' system.

» Are you eating enough fibre (see page 175)? A recent study by Monash University, Australia, showed eating two kiwi fruits a day for four weeks made a difference to people with constipation – increasing frequency and colonic transit time (the speed at which food passes through your lower bowel). Eat the skin, if possible, for maximum benefits.

» How much movement do you do? Sometimes you have to move to 'move'. A brisk walk first thing, especially after a coffee, can help to bring on what's known as a 'mass movement' (bowel movement).

» Are you taking iron supplements? Some – ferrous sulphate – can be very hard on the gut (see page 195).

» Abdominal massage can be very effective. Follow the diagram below either in the morning before you get up or at night lying on your bed.

» How's your gut health overall? For more of a spotlight, see Chapter 12.

Fatigue

Before looking at your diet and energy levels, first get your ferritin (stored iron), folate (B9) and B12 levels checked, especially if you're suffering from heavy periods (or have done in the past) or eat a vegetarian or vegan diet. And while you're at it, ask for a thyroid check as low thyroid can cause extreme tiredness, constipation, hair loss and many of the other symptoms that we commonly associate with perimenopause.

Iron is needed to transport oxygen around your body. If your level is low, it can affect your energy, sleep and fitness

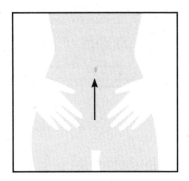

Using massage oil, stroke upwards from the pelvis to the ribcage with flat hands 8–10 times.

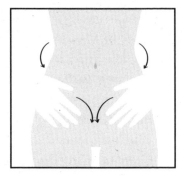

Place both hands on the small of your back. Bring your hands around the top of each hip and down both sides towards your groin. Repeat 10 times.

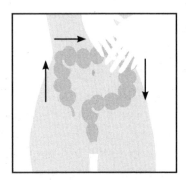

Using both hands on top of each other and starting at the lower right groin, spend a couple of minutes stroking firmly up your right side, across and down your left side, following the direction of your large intestine.

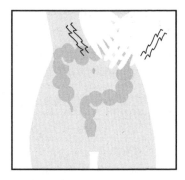

With one hand on top of the other and following your large intestine again, gently push into your abdomen making small shakes with your hands to release gas. Repeat for about a minute.

ABDOMINAL MASSAGE

performance. Too high can affect heart health. Long-term insufficiency might mean you develop iron-deficiency anaemia, symptoms of which include:

» Tiredness
» Shortness of breath
» Heart palpitations
» Pins and needles
» Difficulty concentrating
» Headaches and dizziness
» Sore mouth and tongue
» Hair loss/thinning
» Brittle nails

Your doctor can arrange for blood tests to check your iron and ferritin levels. Ask for a copy of the results. You can be 'in range', but still have a very low score, especially when you consider the 'normal' range for many labs can go as low as 20ng/mL (many healthcare practitioners would consider 19ng/mL to be suggestive of anaemia).

Iron deficiency is best assessed using serum ferritin and an optimal result would be above 80ng/mL. Many women find prescribed iron tablets such as ferrous sulphate upset their gut health, turn their stools black, dry and clay-like and make them constipated. One way round this might be to use an iron spray or patch, which bypasses the gut and is absorbed under the tongue or through the skin.

The daily recommended intake of dietary iron for women under 50 years old is 15mg. Iron-rich foods include liver, lean red meat, chicken, fish and eggs.

You can also get iron from plant-based sources, but it's harder to absorb. Try lentils and beans, tofu, dark green leafy vegetables (spinach, kale, seaweed, watercress, collard greens), parsley, fortified cereals (check labels), and dried fruits like figs and apricots.

Your daily intake of iron might look something like this:

» Two eggs on wholemeal toast
» Beef lasagne + green salad + nuts and seeds
» Mixed bean curry + jacket potato
» 3–4 dried apricots

Other factors to consider:

Tannins from tea, coffee and red wine can affect the absorption of iron (and iron supplements), so avoid drinking them an hour before or after an iron-rich meal or supplement. Zinc supplements can also impede the amount of iron you absorb. Try taking your iron first thing in the morning and your zinc just before bedtime. Vitamin C can help the absorption of iron, so include things like peppers with a steak or squeeze lemon juice over a green leafy salad. Oxalates found in spinach, and phytates found in nuts, grains and legumes, might impact the amount of iron and other nutrients like calcium that your body can extract from foods, although studies are inconclusive. This is one reason why some people sprout or soak nuts, chickpeas and beans.

If you enjoy spinach in your smoothies on a regular basis, try looking for 'baby' (i.e very young) varieties as they have fewer oxalates, or alternatively, look to other greens like kale, romaine lettuce, chard, rocket, parsley, bok choi and celery leaves. Finally, it's worth noting fad diets that involve eliminating carbohydrates and fasting and skipping meals can make you feel really depleted and tired. Work on balancing your plate using the Key 3 approach (see page 182), improving your sleep (see Chapter 8) and improving your gut health (see Chapter 12) to optimise nutrient absorption and energy levels.

Headaches and migraines

Women are three times more likely than men to suffer from headaches and migraines. While we don't know exactly why, there's a lot pointing at hormones – in particular, reduced oestrogen. Women who have never experienced migraines before suddenly start experiencing them during perimenopause and previous sufferers often find they come back with a vengeance, increasing in frequency and intensity.

Try:

» Keeping a food diary to pinpoint any triggers: chocolate and caffeine are common culprits (although it's worth noting for some women caffeine helps as it narrows the dilated blood vessels that can develop with migraines) or track episodes on an app like Migraine Buddy.
» Staying really well hydrated.
» Being vigilant about stabilising your blood-glucose levels (see page 160).
» Taking up to 400mg of magnesium glycinate across the day (talk to a nutritionist about the possibility of a more therapeutic – i.e. larger – dose).
» Talking to your doctor about the possibility of a melatonin prescription. It has been shown to relieve the pain and reduce the frequency of migraines.
» Limiting your alcohol intake: it's a well-known trigger.
» Seeing a craniosacral therapist or physio – working on your neck posture can help.

» Reducing the likelihood of hot flushes (see below) as they've been likened to migraine events, due to their link with stress and cortisol.

» Researching CoQ10. Studies show that 150mg per day can reduce the frequency of migraines by up to 50 per cent.

» Increasing B2-rich (riboflavin) foods: lean meat, eggs, lentils, nuts, green leafy vegetables and dairy, or considering a supplement of 200mg twice a day, which improves the function of an enzyme called MTHFR, which has been linked to migraines.

» Seeing if there's a link with histamine intolerance (see page 208).

» Botox was licensed specifically for the treatment of chronic migraine in 2010. When injected strategically across the scalp and around the brow and eyes, it can have life-changing effects for sufferers. You will need to make sure that the practitioner is trained in accordance with the PREEMPT protocol.

Heavy periods (menorrhagia)

Changes in periods – lighter, heavier, more erratic, spotting – can be one of the first telltale signs you're entering peri-menopause. Heavy periods are debilitating, not to mention traumatic, especially if they result in flooding. Get your iron levels checked (see page 193) as heavy bleeding can lower levels and, weirdly, low iron can actually make periods heavier; one of the many double-edged swords of perimenopause.

Other conditions that can cause heavy bleeding (and which should be discussed with a doctor in the first instance) are:

» Hypothyroidism (low thyroid).
» Fibroids (non-cancerous growths in the uterus).

» Endometriosis (where tissue similar to the lining of the womb starts to grow in other places, such as the ovaries and fallopian tubes).

» Adenomyosis (a condition where the inner lining of the uterus breaks through the wall of the uterus).

» Uterine polyps (small growths attached to the lining of the uterus).

Things to try:

» Reduce or eliminate alcohol, as it can lower progesterone and increase oestrogen (both triggers for heavy periods), as well as spike blood sugar.

» Check your digestion is optimal to ensure oestrogen is being safely excreted out of your body (see Chapter 12).

» Eat two portions of phytoestrogen foods a day (see page 200).

» Keep blood sugar nice and steady to avoid insulin resistance, which can impact ovulation and lower progesterone (see page 160).

» Talk to your doctor about medications: HRT, tranexamic acid and the Mirena coil are commonly used to help with heavy periods.

» Eat more B vitamins, especially B6, which supports progesterone production. Find it in chicken, turkey, oats, bananas, tofu and sweet potatoes.

» Get plenty of greens on your plate as they are power-houses for periods and hormones: broccoli, kale, spinach, romaine lettuce, rocket, spring greens, Swiss chard.

Hot flushes and night sweats (vasomotor symptoms)

There's no magic food that will stop flushes and sweats (HRT is first-line therapy – see Chapter 4), but there are foods and lifestyle factors that make them worse. The most common triggers are alcohol, spicy food, caffeine, stress and smoking. Phytoestrogens – particularly in the early stages of perimenopause – might help, though. The two most studied phytoestrogens are isoflavones (found mostly in soya) and lignans (mostly found in plant-based foods like flaxseeds and legumes), which both have a very mild oestrogenic effect in the body. How so? The truth is, we don't fully know; they seem to have the dual ability to block some oestrogen receptors and turn on others. What we do know is that in a 2016 meta-analysis (where the results of lots of high-quality studies are pooled together) of over 6,000 women, isoflavones were shown to moderately reduce the frequency of hot flushes in some women (though interestingly not night sweats), but the results were far from conclusive.

According to the British Dietetic Association (BDA), 40mg of isoflavones (equal to a palm-sized block of tempeh plus four tablespoons of soya nuts and a glass of soya milk) *may* help reduce the frequency of hot flushes by 20 per cent and severity by 26 per cent. The good news in all this is it's very easy and safe to include phytoestrogens in your diet as they're found in so many foods. Try adding at least two portions a day from the list below. Bear in mind it can take two to three months for the benefits of phytoestrogens to be felt and they seem to work better for some women than others, possibly due to differences in gut bacteria, so they're certainly not a replacement for hormone therapy and it's not a given that they will keep vasomotor symptoms at bay.

There has been a lot of controversy around soya and breast cancer in the past, which understandably has made many women nervous. For the latest research, see the box on page 203.

Phytoestrogen foods:

» Edamame beans
» Soya nuts (roasted edamame beans, often sold in health-food shops as snacks)
» Tofu
» Soya products (milk, yoghurt, etc)
» Tempeh
» Miso
» Natto (a traditional Japanese dish made from fermented soy beans, which is stocked in many supermarkets)
» Soya protein powder
» Flaxseeds
» Chickpeas
» Sesame seeds
» Pistachios

Easy ways to eat more phytoestrogens

» Add 1–2 tablespoons of ground flaxseeds (grind in a NutriBullet or coffee grinder and store in the fridge) to porridge, soups and smoothies.
» Snack on edamame beans. Look for them in the frozen aisle of your supermarket. Steam for 5 minutes and then sprinkle over toppings, such as sea salt, sesame seeds, soy sauce, garlic granules or chilli flakes.
» Make your own hummus. All you need is chickpeas, olive oil, tahini, garlic, lemon juice and a good blender.
» Add roasted chickpeas to salads, stir fries and soups. Drain and rinse a tin of chickpeas. Pat dry with a piece of kitchen paper and spread on a baking tray. Drizzle

with olive oil, salt and maybe some paprika or cumin. Roast in a 200°C oven for 20 minutes or until crispy.

» Swap your normal yoghurt for soya yoghurt. As far as plant-based protein sources go, it's the most similar profile we have to cow's dairy.

» Try scrambling tofu instead of eggs. Don't knock it 'til you've tried it! It's versatile, filling and super-easy.

» Add 2 tablespoons of silken tofu to smoothies: it's creamy, tasteless and full of protein.

» Cut a block of tempeh into cubes; roll in a mix of olive oil, flour, garlic granules and paprika. Oven bake at 180°C for about 25 minutes.

» Add soya nuts (roasted soya beans) to salads and stir-fries or add them to your list of useful snack ideas. You can buy bags of them in most health-food stores.

Soya foods go beyond simply providing phytoestrogens. They also help:

» Reduce cholesterol
» Lower the risk of heart disease
» Improve bone density
» Provide a good source of 'complete' protein

Caution: soya can interfere with the absorption of thyroid medications. Always take your medication on an empty stomach and wait at least four hours until you eat any soya-based foods. If you need added guidance, talk to your doctor.

Other things to consider for hot flushes are:

» Deep, slow breathing (in through the nose and out through the mouth) has been shown to help with temperature control: check out the breathing exercise on page 249 and make sure to implement it the minute you feel a hot flush coming on, as prevention is often better than cure when it comes to hot flushes.

» Acupuncture (see page 260).

The latest on soya and breast cancer

A cursory glance on the internet throws up hundreds of studies, both advocating and vilifying soya. Most of the controversy around soya is based on animal studies and high doses of pure isofla-vones. When we look at the main body of quality human trials, soya does not increase breast cancer risk (and that includes women who have already had breast cancer), which has led to the World Cancer Research Fund concluding that soya foods, consumed as part of a balanced diet, are safe. We'd recommend opting for minimally processed or fermented sources where possible, such as tempeh. If you have breast cancer or have had it in the past, it is always best to follow your oncologist's advice.

Caution: isoflavone supplements have had mixed results and the current advice is to avoid them if you're taking Tamoxifen.

Insomnia

See Chapter 8.

Joint pain

Some points to consider when you have aching muscles and joints, which can feel like they come out of nowhere during perimenopause:

» Motion is lotion when it comes to joints, so even though you might feel achy and stiff, try to keep moving. Walking, yoga and Pilates are all good options.

» Stay hydrated (yep, it's true, there's not much water doesn't help with).

» Try taking a magnesium bisglycinate supplement (400mg daily).

» Follow a Mediterranean diet (see page 166) for its anti-inflammatory benefits.

» Make sure you're taking at least 10mcg of vitamin D in supplement form daily (see Chapter 14).

» Research on curcumin (an anti-inflammatory agent derived from turmeric) as a treatment for inflammatory joint conditions, such as osteoarthritis, is looking promising, though more studies are needed to reach a concrete conclusion. Sadly, your daily turmeric latte is a long way off the therapeutic doses used in the trials, which were between 200–1,000mg/day. To reach those levels, you'll need to invest in a supplement.

» Aim for more Omega 3 than Omega 6 foods to keep inflammation levels in check or supplement to ensure you're getting enough (see Chapter 14).

» If symptoms persist, talk to your doctor to rule out other, more serious conditions.

» There is some evidence supporting the use of collagen supplements for reducing joint pain from exercise or osteoarthritis.

» Supplementing with vitamin C may play a role in recovery from joint injuries. Try taking 500mg a day for a therapeutic dose.

Low bone density

Future-proofing your bone health is vital at every stage of life (you actually reach peak bone mass in your late 20s), not least during perimenopause. Bone stores start depleting as we hit our 30s and then accelerate quite alarmingly as we hit our 40s, dialling up the risk of osteoporosis (brittle bones) and fractures in later life. In terms of dietary considerations, the obvious one is calcium, but there are other minerals and nutrients you will need to include alongside it. Also see page 238 and the importance of resistance/strength training exercise for bone health in Chapter 13.

Nutrients for strong bones

Calcium: the recommended dose is 700mg daily if you're under 50 and 1,200mg if you're over 50. You should be able to get it from your diet: dairy, fortified plant milk, green leafy vegetables, tofu (make sure it says 'calcium set' on the label), seeds, beans, lentils and bread. Avoid calcium supplements (unless prescribed by your doctor) as in large amounts they can increase the likelihood of kidney stones and harden the wall of your arteries.

Protein: see page 169 for recommended amounts.
Vitamin D: see page 256 for supplementation advice.

Magnesium, zinc, boron, vitamin K and selenium are also essential. There are many supplements that combine all these nutrients into one bone-friendly capsule.

240mg of calcium looks like . . .

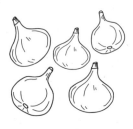

5 dried figs

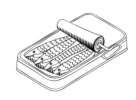

½ can (60g) sardines

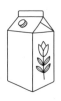

200ml fortified plant milk

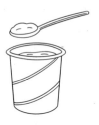

150g natural yoghurt

30g hard cheese

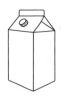

200ml cow's milk

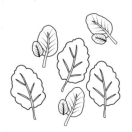

8 tbsp steamed kale

75g tofu

(check label that it's 'calcium set')

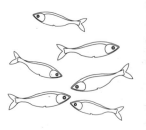

35g whitebait

CALCIUM

Other considerations
Weight-bearing exercise is essential for strong bones. Walking counts and dancing is good, but the gold standard is anything that involves jumping, so think volleyball, a vigorous game of tennis, netball, martial arts and box jumping (usually done in HIIT classes). Start small and build up. Skipping, running and jogging are all good options too, whereas swimming and cycling aren't as they don't offer enough impact.

Things to be aware of
Smoking decreases bone density by up to 25 per cent.

Oxalates in raw spinach bind to calcium and impede its absorption. Avoid daily raw spinach for this reason (NB. baby or young spinach has fewer oxalates) or lightly steam/wilt to break the oxalates down.

You can check your existing bone density via a DEXA scan. It's highly unlikely that you'll get one through the NHS, although you have a strong argument if you went through early menopause. If not, you'll have to be referred or pay to go privately.

Skin issues

Skin issues and perimenopause seem to go hand in hand. Hormones, stress, poor sleep, alcohol, histamine intolerance and a less than brilliant diet might all play a role.

Dry skin

A balanced diet should always be a priority when it comes to hormonal skin issues to ensure you're nourishing your skin from the inside out, but it's not a magic formula.

There are some no-brainers to bear in mind: cut back on fried food, refined sugars and ultra-processed foods (foods that have been processed in some way and contain additives, colouring and preservatives), and hydrate well. Consider taking an Omega 3 supplement (see Chapter 14) to help with hydration.

Other points to bear in mind:

» Make room for healthy fats, like avocados, oily fish (see page 172), olive oil, and nuts and seeds.
» Balanced blood sugar (see page 160) is vital for healthy skin. Long-term glucose in the blood is associated with advanced glycation end products (AGEs), which have been shown to damage collagen and increase skin ageing.
» Despite their popularity, collagen supplements haven't been shown to improve collagen levels in skin. Collagen is simply broken down when ingested and used by the body where it's deemed most important – i.e. you can't direct it to your crow's feet, sadly. The UK Advertising Standards Authority (ASA) has criticised ads suggesting collagen contributes to youthful skin, due to the lack of evidence.
» Vitamin D supports skin cell turnover and has been linked to improvements in conditions like dry skin, psoriasis and eczema. For dosages and preparations, go to page 256.
» Try taking an Omega 7 supplement for three months (also known as Sea Buckthorn Oil) and/or a good-quality, low molecular weight oral hyaluronic acid. Both work on hydrating and locking in moisture into cells, which is why they're also linked with possibly alleviating osteoarthritis, dry eyes and vaginal dryness.

Histamine intolerance, itchy skin and hormones

Histamine – a chemical found naturally in the body – is a crucial part of your immune system. It's part of the inflammatory response that helps clear irritants (such as pollen) and invaders from the body, but also plays an important role in the production of stomach acid and digestion. In the right amounts, histamine is vital to wellbeing, but when it doesn't get cleared from the body and builds up it can be problematic.

Many women find histamine intolerance becomes very pronounced when hormones are fluctuating. There are a few mechanisms at play, but the most significant is that oestrogen stimulates histamine and vice versa, so if oestrogen levels are peaking – highly possible if you're perimenopausal – you may well feel the effects of histamine.

High histamine symptoms mimic allergy reactions (it's sometimes referred to as a 'pseudo allergy') and include itchy skin and eyes, runny nose, sensitivity to allergens like pollen, heat intolerance, rosacea symptoms worsening, headaches, migraines, hives, rashes, palpitations, joint aches, dizziness, IBS and nausea. Symptoms tend to come and go. In addition, some women find allergies and intolerances that haven't affected them for years suddenly resurface around their perimenopause years, which may well be due to histamine.

There are three things to consider if you think you might be having problems with histamine:

1. Some foods are high in histamine and others trigger histamine to be released in the body. See the list below for some of the most high-histamine foods, but bear in mind you may have a very different looking list as reactions to histamine are so individual. Histamine levels in food can vary depending on age, storage and processing.
    »   Aged cheeses (like parmesan)
    »   Bone broth
    »   Cured meats: salami, ham, sausages
    »   Smoked and tinned fish

» Shellfish
» Citrus fruits: oranges, limes, lemons, grapefruits
» Other fruits: bananas, papaya, pineapple, strawberries, kiwi
» Vegetables: aubergine, tomatoes, spinach, avocado, rocket, mushrooms, canned vegetables
» Dark chocolate
» Fermented foods: kefir, sauerkraut, yoghurt, kombucha
» Alcohol
» Leftovers (food that's not fresh)
» Nuts/seeds that have been stored for a long time
» Dairy (sheep's, goat's or A2 cow's milk are often better tolerated)
» Vinegar
» Yeast
» Black and green tea

2. DAO (diamine oxidase) – an enzyme produced naturally in the gut – breaks histamine down once it has done its job. Sometimes women have low levels or have problems making enough. Much of your DAO enzyme is made in the intestinal lining, so gut health and stress reduction both play a big role in histamine reduction.

Tips:

» To make DAO, you need good levels of copper (liver, shiitake mushrooms, leafy greens, oysters), vitamin C (250mg taken in 3–4 doses throughout the day) and all the B vitamins, but especially B6. You can also buy DAO in supplement form but it is expensive. Take 30 minutes before a meal that includes histamine-rich foods.
» Magnesium (see page 253) is also important.

» L-glutamine (500mg a day) and Quercetin (500mg twice a day) both block the action of histamine. You can buy them in supplement form.

» Good gut bacteria break down histamine (see Chapter 12).

» Regulating progesterone (via HRT) can help to counterbalance the histamine-producing effects of oestrogen, but HRT also increases oestrogen, potentially fuelling histamine intolerance symptoms further. Every woman responds individually. Many histamine intolerance symptoms cross over with those of perimenopause, which can be very confusing. If you think you have a histamine intolerance, make sure you flag it up to your doctor when discussing HRT. If necessary, look at www.histamineintolerance.org.uk and print off any relevant information to back up your case.

» Alcohol, antidepressants and painkillers, like ibuprofen, can reduce your body's ability to break down histamine.

» Histamine intolerance tests are notoriously unreliable.

» Diet should always be addressed first, but there are over-the-counter medications (antihistamines) and prescription drugs (H2 blockers) that can help.

» Some women have a genetic variant (AOC1), which means they're more predisposed to histamine intolerance (this will show up on DNA tests).

3. Try keeping a symptom diary to identify your triggers, or work on an elimination diet alongside a nutritionist. For more information about histamine intolerance, visit www.histamineintolerance.org.uk.

Acne

Perhaps one of the most visible similarities between puberty and perimenopause is on the skin. Hormones are running wild and skin becomes oily, blemish-prone and hard to manage, just like it might have done in teenage years. Congested skin can make an already stressful time even harder and lots of women feel ashamed at not having clear skin.

If you're an acne sufferer, we can almost guarantee you've tried (or someone has suggested) cutting out dairy. For a small subset of women this works, so is worth exploring, but for the majority it doesn't have much effect. Acne in perimenopause is usually due to androgenic (male) hormones like testosterone which, when oestrogen and progesterone dip, become dominant. This is often the case in women who have PCOS (polycystic ovarian syndrome) and is also fairly common among perimenopausal women whose hormones are unstable. As always, a balanced whole foods-based diet (i.e. one not reliant on processed foods) with plenty of fruit and vegetables and lots of water is advised. Gut health is also key (see Chapter 12). We think refined high-sugar foods might play a role in driving acne and that foods rich in zinc, such as shellfish, eggs, pumpkin seeds, chickpeas and beans, or a three-month course of 10mg zinc daily, may have an anti-inflammatory effect. But this is not a magic bullet.

If your spots are getting you down, the most effective thing you can do is look to your skincare (see page 78) and, possibly, prescribed medication creams/gels such as adapalene, duac or a course of antibiotics such as lymecycline or erythromycin. Or talk to your doctor about spironolactone (an anti-androgen) or in more severe cases oral isotretinoin (Roaccutane), for which you'll need to see a dermatologist.

Thinning hair

Because hair is not an essential tissue, it's the last part of you to receive nutrients, and the first to be withheld from them, so any nutritional deficiency – even a small one – can negatively impact your hair. Eating at least a palm-sized portion of protein (which is what your hair is made of), alongside a serving of complex carbohydrates will provide your hair with the energy it needs to grow. Likewise, iron is also essential.

The supplement that usually gets cited with hair loss is vitamin B7, otherwise known as biotin. Evidence is scant, although anecdotally women find it helpful. It's worth noting that biotin supplements have more substantial results for brittle nails, so if that's an issue for you and you're noticing hair changes it could be worthwhile investing in a biotin supplement. If not, you can get biotin from lots of food sources, including edamame beans, eggs, almonds, oats, cauliflower and bananas.

Lifestyle considerations:

» Aggressive styling and heated appliances can be very damaging to hair.
» Try not to pull hair back too tightly; use soft hair ties that don't snag.
» Try a 5-minute scalp massage at night.
» Minoxidil (also known as Regaine) is an over-the-counter medication that stimulates growth by encouraging blood flow to the follicles. It is backed by robust clinical data, but only works as long as you use it.
» Viviscal is a supplement backed by several clinical trials that treats hair loss and accelerates growth. Results can take six months to show so you'll need considerable patience – and a healthy budget – to see the rewards.
» Be gentle when towel drying, brushing and detangling hair.
» Newer treatment options out there are micro-needling, PRP (platelet-rich protein) and growth factor serums,

for which more data is needed before we can give them a definitive thumbs up.

Vaginal dryness

Unfortunately, no food is going to cure vaginal dryness. Your first port of call in this instance should be localised oestrogen (see page 29), which is safe and extremely effective. From a dietary viewpoint, keep an eye on your hydration and make sure you're including lots of healthy fats in your diet.

Just as your facial skin needs collagen for support, moisture and volume, so do the tissues of your vagina. Vitamin C, adequate protein, zinc and vitamin E all play an important role. In terms of supplements, a small study of 116 women showed an improvement in vaginal moisture levels from taking 3g of Sea Buckthorn Oil (Omega 7) daily for three months.

The bottom line

» The foods you eat can have a marked impact on your perimenopause symptoms.
» Include the Key 3 – protein, fibre, fats – to help prevent anxiety and mood swings.
» Your brain is 60 per cent fat, so enjoy healthy fats like nuts, seeds and avocados.
» Stay hydrated – just a 1 per cent drop in hydration can affect your brain's ability to think straight and perform well.
» Get your ferritin (iron) levels checked, especially if you're tired, have palpitations, suffer from repeated mouth ulcers or have thinning hair.

»   Keep a symptom diary to work out migraine triggers or use an app like Migraine Buddy.

»   The most common stimulants for hot flushes are caffeine, alcohol, stress, spicy food and smoking.

»   Are you eating enough calcium? You need 700mg a day for good bone health if you're under 50 and 1,200mg a day if you're over 50.

CHAPTER 12

Clever Guts

It's hard to overstate how important good gut bacteria are to your health.

Gut health has gone from a trending topic to a fully paid-up, integral part of accepted medicine. There's now no doubt in anyone's mind the good bacteria that reside in your digestive tract are inextricably linked to wellbeing and good health. But what influence does the gut have on perimenopause symptoms? More than you might expect. In this chapter we'll take a look at the plethora of tasks your gut – and its resident microbes – do for you and your hormones, and how to optimise them through easy-to-implement diet and lifestyle strategies.

You see, the gut isn't just about how much and how well you digest and absorb nutrients from food – though this in itself is crucial for things like energy, heart health and clear skin. Your gut is also responsible for clearing out old hormones, making certain vitamins, defending against potentially harmful pathogens, as well as influencing mood, brain function and even weight. When you check out the overwhelming evidence now emerging, it's hard to over-state how important good gut bacteria are to your health.

What even is 'the gut'?

The gut is a 9-metre tube that runs from entry (mouth) to exit (bum). It houses trillions of bacteria, fungi and viruses (known as the microbiota), mainly in the large intestine. These tiny tenants earn their keep by supporting your physical and mental health in myriad ways; telling you when you're hungry, fighting infection, making vitamin K and B12, influencing GABA – the neurotransmitter that helps you feel calm – and even dictating how much of your medication is absorbed. So, naturally, we want to help our gut microbes thrive at all costs. But how?

Keeping it in check

Although the gut is remarkably complex, we have the ability to influence it through what we eat and how we live. As a perimenopausal woman facing a maelstrom of symptoms, this is good news; finally, an aspect of your health that's within your control. Even better news – small changes can have a dramatic effect in improving the state of your gut. In fact, in some cases, good gut bacteria can be increased in a matter of days following a change of diet. But when the microbiota becomes imbalanced and levels of bad bacteria outweigh the good – i.e through long-term alcohol or antibiotic use – it can lead to hormonal disturbances and inflammation.

Gut health and perimenopause symptoms

Gut health is a big topic and, to be honest, scientists are only just scratching the surface when it comes to the research. To narrow it down to the areas that might be affecting you, let's look at the five most important reasons to look after gut health during perimenopause.

1. Brain health

The gut and brain are connected via the vagus nerve, a long two-way communication channel that runs from our brain stem down through our diaphragm into our gut. Think of it as a fibre-optic cable enabling the brain and the gut to talk to each other (known as the gut-brain axis). It is, we think, part of the reason we feel butterflies when we're excited or might have to dash to the toilet when we're nervous or stressed. The connection is so tightly interwoven that the gut is sometimes called the second brain and scientists believe conditions like anxiety, depression and dementia, which we have always assumed start in the brain, can actually be linked to the gut.

2. Mood

While we're only just working out the links between gut health and mood, we know for sure around 90 per cent of our happy neurotransmitter, serotonin, is produced and stored in the gut. Even though serotonin in the gut can't cross through into the brain, scientists think it has a strong influence elsewhere in the body. Studies show that some gut bacteria strains help with the production of tryptophan (see page 135) the precursor to serotonin, so it's becoming clearer than ever our good gut bugs play a crucial role in how happy and content we feel.

3. Oestrogen balance

The bacteria in your gut might play a part in circulating oestrogen levels. Scientists think the estrobolome is a collection of bacteria that helps regulate the amount of oestrogen in the body. The suggestion is that imbalances in these bacteria might cause either a deficiency or an excess of free oestrogen, which can potentially give rise to oestrogen-related health issues such as endometriosis, PCOS and possibly breast cancer. Researchers think the estrobolome might also have an influence on perimenopause symptoms like weight, mood swings and libido.

Emerging research points towards good gut health potentially playing a part in excreting metabolised oestrogen via your stool. Stool is made up of many things, including undigested food (fibre), toxins and, in the case of pre-menopausal and possibly perimenopausal women, oestrogen. The hypothesis is that if you don't excrete this oestrogen effectively (e.g. if you suffer long-term constipation or gut health issues) it can get reabsorbed into the body. This could potentially lead to symptoms of oestrogen dominance. The evidence isn't categorical and further studies are needed to assess the exact relationship between the gut microbiota and circulating oestrogen, particularly in the case of reducing hormone-driven breast cancer risk in post-menopausal women. Nonetheless, one thing is clear: fibre is extremely beneficial for women's hormone health.

4. Immune health

Between 70 and 80 per cent of your immune system is located in the wall linings of your gut. These cells act like bouncers, refusing entry to potential toxins and letting in the proteins and molecules your body actually needs. Sometimes this process goes awry, leading to allergies and autoimmune conditions such as Hashimoto's (where your immune system attacks your thyroid) and coeliac disease, leading some researchers to believe there's an overlap between gut dysfunction and these types of conditions. The exact mechanism is unclear, but we do know there's a marked increase in autoimmune diseases and allergies in women around the time of perimenopause, possibly due to oestrogen's effects on the microbiota.

5. Weight

Many studies appear to link low gut bacteria diversity with obesity, reduced insulin sensitivity and increased body weight.

Although we don't know the full picture yet, we think it's partly down to the gut's role in producing chemicals, like butyrate, acetate, peptide YY and GLP-1, which tell your brain when you're hungry and when you're full. The natural conclusion suggests improving your gut flora might well help with weight loss. So far the research points towards certain strains of bacteria being associated with weight management. *Prevotella* and *Akkermansia* are the ones we know most about, although it should be noted most of the studies have been done on mice not humans. It's not currently possible to bottle these strains, so we need to get them from food. *Prevotella* is associated with plant-rich diets (in particular complex carbs, fruit and vegetables) and *Akkermansia* enjoy feasting on Omega 3 and fruits such as cranberries, grapes, pomegranates, raspberries and aronia berry juice. When it comes to gut health, though, all plant foods are welcome – the more diverse, the better.

Small changes, big results

The good news is that it's possible to change your microbiota over the course of just a few days. We're talking small changes here, not a complete diet overhaul. Our advice is to do whatever feels realistic for you right now – choose just one or two changes from the list below; once they're bedded in and part of everyday life, choose your next goal. And if it all just feels like too much right now, simply try to have a couple more portions of vegetables and fruit this week and come back and take another look below when you're in a better place.

Prebiotics at a glance
Prebiotics are fibres (from plants) that your gut microbes feed on. The best-known prebiotics are inulin, FOS (fructo oligosaccharides) and GOS

(galacto oligosaccharides) and you'll find them in a vast number of vegetables, fruits, grains and even things like fennel tea. This is just another of the many arguments for increasing the number and diversity of plant-based foods into your overall diet. You can buy prebiotic supplements, but the most effective way to increase prebiotics is simply to eat them. Here's a list of the big hitters:

» Jerusalem artichokes
» Onions
» Leeks
» Okra
» Garlic
» Mushrooms
» Chicory root
» Beetroot
» Asparagus
» Bananas (the greener, the better)
» Apricots
» Nectarines
» Pomegranate
» Sharon fruit
» Fennel and fennel tea
» Nuts (almonds, cashews, hazelnuts, pistachios)
» Grains (oats, rye, spelt, sourdough)
» Pulses (lentils, butterbeans, chickpeas)

If you're up for the challenge, here are eight ways you could go about improving your gut:

1. Eat more plants

The American Gut Project found people who consumed at least 30 different plant types a week had more diverse gut bacteria. And, remember, more microbes can mean better oestrogen balance, stronger immunity, improved skin health, more efficient nutrient absorption and better blood-sugar control. Music to perimenopausal ears.

The last one is especially important as blood-sugar balance (see page 160) has a knock-on effect with mood, energy and cravings. Don't get too hung up on the numbers though: 30 is a guide, it's not the law. All fruit, vegetables, herbs, spices, nuts, seeds and wholegrains count towards your total. Try noting them down on your phone. Get the family involved too. Breakfast is a great opportunity to get your numbers up. If you start the day with porridge oats, blueberries, sunflower seeds and a sprinkle of cinnamon, that's four right there. Just be aware that to increase the diversity (and to keep increasing the numbers), you'll need to mix it up a little across the week, i.e. raspberries and pumpkin seeds one day, strawberries and walnuts the day after, and maybe swap the porridge oats for buckwheat oats or chia seeds the day after that.

2. Make friends with fermented foods

You might not know this, but you've been colonising your gut microbes since the moment you were born. Your birth (vaginal or caesarean), whether you were breast-fed, your lifestyle, environment, medication and even the pets you live with shape the number and different strains of bacteria living in your gut. Antibiotics, alcohol, stress, poor diet, age and lack of sleep can all negatively impact your gut's happiness.

Although the research to date isn't concrete, one way we think you might be able to populate your gut with good microbes is via fermented foods that contain beneficial bacteria similar to those in the gut. Kefir (fermented yoghurt), live yoghurt, miso (a paste made from fermented soybeans), kimchi (spicy, fermented vegetables), sauerkraut (fermented cabbage), kombucha (a kind of fizzy fermented tea), pickles and the Japanese food natto (fermented soybeans with an acquired taste that some liken to Marmite, sold in the frozen section of most supermarkets) are all ways to potentially keep your gut bugs plentiful. Although there's a question mark over just how many microbes reach the gut intact, fermented foods are tasty, affordable (many can be made at home), accessible (look in the chilled aisle of your local supermarket) and harmless.

Make your own cow's milk kefir

You'll need:

2 x 500ml kilner jars

Kefir grains (we like everygoodthing.co.uk but there are lots of sellers online)

1 pint full-fat cow's milk (ideally organic)

Small sieve or strainer

Add 1 teaspoon of kefir grains to one of your glass jars and top with the milk. Pop the lid on and leave in a warm place to ferment (an airing cupboard works well). After 24 hours the milk should be looking firmer and more 'set', strain the liquid using a small sieve or strainer (keep the grains as you're going to be using them again) into the second jar or bottle. This is your kefir! It'll keep for around 7 days in the fridge.

Clean the jar you used to ferment the grains, pop the grains back in, refill with a fresh pint of milk and you're ready to make your next batch. If you ever need a break or are going away, donate the grains to someone else. They can give them back on your return! Alternatively, just top the grains with a little milk and store in the fridge for up to 7 days until you're ready to start fermenting again. You may notice that the grains start growing after a few rounds of fermentation. This is good, it means they're happy. When they've doubled in size, give half of them away to a friend or freeze them for later use.

A note on taste: kefir is an acquired taste and quite different to the ones you find in shops. Mix into smoothies, overnight oats or chia pudding. It's fine to sweeten to taste using a little honey or maple syrup.

If you're new to fermented foods or have IBS-type symptoms, start with a tablespoon a day and build up to about 150ml.

3. Put more prebiotics on your plate

Prebiotics are the food – mainly fibre – your gut microbes eat. You'll find them in thousands of plant-based foods (see box). Eating plenty of different types of fibre will help your microbes colonise and thrive. As with everything fibre related, start low and slow and build up your tolerance. Inulin – a type of prebiotic found in chicory root – has been linked to how well you produce the hormone ghrelin, which tells you how hungry you are, and leptin, which signals when you've had enough to eat. As you'd expect, both hormones play a critical role in healthy weight management. Inulin comes in 250g bags online, and can be added to porridge, smoothies or hot drinks; it has a slightly sweet taste.

4. Rest your microbiome

Even with the best diet in the world, poor sleep has been shown to impact the biodiversity of your gut. So rather than spending money on supplements and artisan-brewed kombucha, your first port of call should be looking at the quality and quantity of your sleep. Disturbed sleep impacts your gut bacteria's natural rhythm and studies show just two days of getting less sleep than you need impacts their wellbeing substantially. Poor sleep can also raise inflammation levels, which may well translate to increased gut disorders like IBS and acid reflux. Sleep is thought to be bi-directional, i.e. lack of sleep impacts gut microbes and imbalanced microbes seem to negatively impact sleep. See Chapter 8 for advice on getting better shut eye.

Another way to rest and improve your microbiota is through fasting. We're not talking about anything hard-core, simply having a 12-hour period (including overnight) of not eating. Fasting has been shown to help increase *Akkermansia* – the microbe associated with weight and better insulin sensitivity – and to improve reflux symptoms.

5. Dial down stress

Lots of women find their digestive health takes a bit of a nosedive when hormones are playing up. One of oestrogen's many jobs is to keep cortisol levels low, so when oestrogen levels dip, cortisol – and stress – can rise. This means a slowing down of the digestive process, which can be exacerbated further if you happen to be taking iron, thyroid medication or anti-depressants. High levels of cortisol mean your body will automatically put digestion lower down on the priority list, thus heightening digestive disorders and making your life (and potentially those around you) uncomfortable. It's worth remembering that caffeine and alcohol can worsen stress, while exercise and movement can help (see Chapter 13).

6. Be mindful of additives

Although the majority of artificial sweeteners and emulsifiers have passed food safety trials, there's still a question over what they do to your gut microbes. Some animal studies point towards sugar substitutes like aspartame, saccharin and sucralose adversely impacting your microbiota. And certain emulsifiers, like carboxymethylcellulose (CMC), polysorbate 80 (P80), guar gum and carrageenan – often found in margarine, processed meats, long-life wraps and bread products – have been linked to damaging the gut wall lining. This doesn't mean they will have the same impact on human health or that all additives are 'bad', but it's worth being aware of the number of additives you consume, and limiting them in your diet if possible. It's also worth noting many gluten-free foods contain emulsifiers to help 'glue' ingredients together. Moral of the story: always read labels carefully.

7. Don't deprive your microbes

It can be very tempting to follow the latest diet that's doing the rounds on social media. But when it comes to your gut microbes, you need to be careful, particularly if you're restricting certain types of foods. The obvious one is carbohydrates. We need quality carbs for a number of gut-related processes, including serotonin production, the neurotransmitter that helps shape our mood and happiness. Carbs are also a very useful source of fibre, which your gut bugs feast on. Hungry gut bacteria aren't productive, don't reproduce and don't have the optimal conditions to thrive. By all means keep a check on the quantity and quality of the carbohydrates you're consuming but, for the sake of your gut, please don't omit them completely.

8. Get wonky

Phytochemicals or plant chemicals have potent antioxidant (disease-fighting) properties that help protect us from cell damage, premature ageing and inflammation. They're what give fruits and vegetables their colour and smell. Wonky fruit and vegetables that are less than perfect in shape and size tend to have higher levels of phytochemicals, so opt for odd shapes when you're doing the weekly shop. Oddbox.co.uk deliver produce supermarkets turn away for being aesthetically unpleasing.

There are thought to be many hundreds of different types of phytochemicals, but the ones we know most about are polyphenols. Polyphenols aren't deemed essential to our diet but they're garnering more and more traction in health and nutrition circles, particularly when it comes to the gut. This is because when our gut bacteria digest polyphenols they produce compounds that can help with everything from improving memory to lowering inflammation. The most common example are polyphenols found in a variety of plant-based foods, including herbs (dried and fresh), spices and dark chocolate.

Best polyphenol foods include sage, thyme, turmeric, ginger, cinnamon, oregano, green tea, black tea, cocoa, red wine, blueberries, blackcurrants, cherries, blackberries, strawberries, raspberries, prunes, apples, flaxseeds, hazelnuts, pecans, almonds, olives, chicory, red onion, spinach, black beans, white beans, broccoli, asparagus and extra virgin olive oil.

Faeces and farts: the facts

We couldn't have a chapter on gut health without talking about poo. Believe it or not, your toilet habits say a lot about your health. Sure, it's not exactly dinner table conversation, but we need to be a little more open to examining our number twos: from colour to consistency. Curious to know more?

» We all fart: 15–20 times a day is totally normal.

» If you increase the amount of fibre you're eating, you may notice more wind. It's just your gut bacteria doing their job.

» Sulphurous (eggy) farts can be a result of high protein (sometimes whey powders can cause wind), cruciferous vegetables (kale, Brussels sprouts, cabbage, broccoli are the most common offenders) or alcohol.

» If you suspect your wind is associated with a food intolerance (i.e. you get symptoms after consuming dairy), seek professional advice.

» Although we often think having a bowel movement once a day is healthy, actually anything from three times a day to three times a week is considered 'normal'. The key is what's normal for you. If bowel habits change (the NHS guidance says for two weeks or longer), it's time to talk to a doctor.

» Stool should be mid- to dark brown and sausage-like. Be aware beetroot will often make stool red and iron supplements can make them black.

» When stressed, your gut function slows down as the body diverts blood supply away from the digestive system. This might mean you get constipated (see page 192). For some people stress can do the opposite, with the increased adrenaline causing diarrhoea.

» There should be a certain post-stool satisfaction, a feeling that you've fully evacuated. For the perfect bowel movement position, sit on the toilet with your knees higher than your hips, perhaps placing your feet on a small stool. If you frequently feel as though there's more to come but it won't come out, it could be due to conditions such as a prolapse. If in doubt, and especially if you have other symptoms, talk to your GP or seek advice from a women's physio.

Red flags ... when to go to doctor:

» Unexplained or prolonged bloating.
» Blood in stool.
» IBS symptoms for longer than two weeks.
» A change in bowel habits.
» Suspected coeliac disease. Note that you need to include gluten in your diet for six weeks prior to testing for coeliac disease.

Probiotic supplements

There's a tendency towards glamorising gut health and feeding into the myth that you need to invest in loads of fancy supplements and expensive probiotics, when often they're unnecessary. In actual fact, clinical data only really supports probiotics in a handful of cases: mainly IBS, traveller's diarrhoea (holiday tum) and after a course of antibiotics. There are lots of different types and formulations, usually in capsule or liquid form. When choosing one, look on the label to check that they contain a large number of CFUs (colony forming units). Ideally you want 10–20 billion, as many will be lost on the way through your digestive tract. Also, check to see if there are independent clinical trials to back up the manufacturer's claims. Some of the more generic, broad spectrum brands, which have had positive results in clinical trials for the symptoms mentioned above, are Aflorex, Symprove, OptiBac, Bio-Kult and VSL#3. Store your probiotic supplements properly; some need to be kept in the fridge, so check the label.

Many clients ask if it's necessary to carry out stool analysis tests for feedback on microbiota diversity. While they're interesting, they're also expensive and, because your gut bacteria can change so quickly, they don't have much longevity. Shifts in your diet mean your test results could look very different if you were to repeat in a week's time.

Probiotics don't work for everyone, but they're generally safe. Try them for 8–12 weeks and keep a diary to note if they improve your symptoms. If they don't, it might be worth trying an alternative route.

Uchenna's story

I'm always on the go and I fly overseas regularly. I eat well and don't drink alcohol, but I've had some mild digestive complaints since I was in my early 20s. When I hit perimenopause though my symptoms turned into full-blown IBS. I've subsequently tried every fad diet and supplement going. My GP gave me Buscopan, which is prescribed for stomach and bladder cramps, but they made me feel really nauseous. I even spent a fortune on a course of colonic cleanses, which were not only incredibly uncomfortable, they actually made things worse.

After one hair-raising dash from a board meeting presentation to the loo, which coincided with a particularly vehement hot flush, I sought nutrition advice and thought she'd take out loads of foods and send me on my way. But in our first session together we didn't even talk about food, we just discussed the connection between stress and IBS. Before that it hadn't dawned on me that my job, and the frantic nature of my life, coupled with the stress of hormonal changes, could be triggering my gut troubles. I've now dialled down my rather high-octane exercise routine as it was an added stressor and added in more low-fi stuff like yoga. I've also had to get comfy with tracking and analysing what comes out in the toilet, but things are definitely better. About three months ago, when things were feeling more settled, I started a capsule probiotic that I take with me when I'm travelling. It has made life infinitely more bearable.

The bottom line

» Small but mighty: boosting your microbes can have massive health-changing benefits.
» Simple is best: fibre, fermented foods, diet diversity, rest, exercise.
» Plant life: the most important thing you can do for your gut is to eat more plants.
» Know your normal: if you notice changes in your bowel habits, talk to a doctor.
» Pills and potions: probiotics are not a 'cure-all', but for most people they're safe to try.
» Odd ones out: fruit and vegetables with unusual lumps and bumps have more polyphenols.

CHAPTER 13

Move Your Body

Your future self is the sum of all the small actions you choose from today.

Did you know physical inactivity is rated just behind smoking when it comes to major contributors to ill health? For lots of perimenopausal women, even though they understand the myriad benefits of moving more, exercise is the first thing to fall by the wayside when they're tired, feeling low or time poor. In this chapter we'll explore the litany of benefits moving your body will bring during this time of life. We'll talk about why we believe weight training should be given out on prescription, how you don't have to be zen to enjoy yoga and how it's never ever too late to start exercising. The beauty of movement is that it doesn't matter what type you choose, it all counts. And you won't regret a minute of it.

There's a significant body of research detailing the effects of exercise on perimenopausal women. We know regular movement helps alleviate stiffness, fatigue, concentration issues, poor sleep and irritability. And although definitive results are inconclusive, a number of studies have shown exercise – in particular, strength training – can lessen the likelihood of having hot flushes, particularly in woman who already have decent levels of fitness.

The short-term benefits of movement include increased endurance, metabolism and energy; healthier muscles, joints and bones; decreased stress; improved cognitive function and better sleep. An impressive list at any time of life, but particularly pertinent for women who are feeling the effects of perimenopause. And the accolades don't end there. Regular long-term exercise is associated with improved outcomes across a number of chronic diseases, including cancer, heart disease, stroke, blood pressure, Type 2 diabetes, obesity, osteoporosis and depression. And if all that isn't enough, Harvard researchers suggest a mere 15 minutes of physical activity a day can add three years to your life span.

If there's one take-home to be had from all this knowledge, it's that physical activity promotes better ageing. It keeps us vital, strong, switched on and reduces our vulnerability to a wide range of diseases, including respiratory infections.

According to the World Health Organization (WHO), 30 minutes of daily physical activity reduces premature death rates by around 20 per cent. In fact, according to WHO, not leading an active life features in the ten leading causes of death. So why are we still such a bunch of refuseniks?

The sticking point for many of us when it comes to exercise is the idea itself. Perhaps the word 'exercise' needs to be reframed. The negative connotations associated with gruelling gym sessions or hours of tedious trudging on a treadmill are entrenched in many of our minds. The added kicker is our high-tech lifestyles mean we don't *need* to be physically active if we don't want to be; we have to *choose* to be. If we want to meet NHS guidelines (see box below) it has to be a concerted effort, which often doesn't come naturally. Here are some ideas on how to shift our mindset and find ways to make exercise more appealing:

» Multi-task: use exercise as a time to educate yourself by listening to podcasts and audio books.
» Music motivates: create playlists that you can't wait to move to.
» Break it up into small chunks throughout the day: 'exercise snacking'.
» Diarise it and treat it as an appointment that cannot be rescheduled.
» Make it social by inviting friends along – this helps with accountability too.
» Choose something you enjoy; there's no one-size-fits-all solution.
» Mix it up with cardio and weighted exercises to keep things fresh.
» Join a running group, sign up to events like parkrun – a free weekly Saturday morning 5K run (or walk), open to people of all ages and abilities, which takes place in local parks – or check out cycling clubs near you.
» If you've never run before, try the free NHS 'Couch to 5K' app.
» Set small daily goals. Lots of scientific data suggests frequency is important.
» Loan a dog from a neighbour or friend or sign up to borrowmydoggy.com.

Don't take it easy as you age

There's a long-held belief that we need to slow down as we move through life and that 'at a certain age' we can't do what we used to do. Not true. The current life expectancy for women is 83, which means we'll hopefully be living half to a third of our lives post-menopausal.

What we do now to optimise our physical wellbeing will have a significant bearing on how strong, fit and flexible we are in the years to come. For anyone worried about having left it too late, check out the social media luminary Joan MacDonald (@trainwithjoan) who embarked on a life-changing fitness journey in her early 70s and is now busting out unassisted pull-ups and lifting barbells. Incidentally, she's also stopped taking her blood pressure, cholesterol and acid reflux medication and lost 27kg in the process. If a woman in her 70s can do this, there's no doubt you can too. It won't happen overnight, but with patience and persistence you will get there. Our advice? Trust the process, but try to enjoy it too, and remember that hard work pays off. Your future self is the sum of all the small actions you choose from today, so let's take a look at a few of those options.

What kind of exercise should we be doing?

The general consensus is anything goes and even the smallest amount is better than nothing. The key is finding something you love doing that doesn't feel like a chore. You're aiming for consistency – keep showing up, keep putting in the work, keep improving – and if you want to smash a few PBs be our guest.

The only caveat, if you're new to exercise, is to ease in gently: without the buffering effects of oestrogen on our muscles, tendons and ligaments, we're more prone to injury.

So, with that in mind, let's take a look at some of the options.

Walking

Walking ticks a lot of boxes. It's free, convenient, easy, safe, doesn't call for any special equipment and you can do it anywhere. We'd go as far as saying it's the most underrated form of exercise going. The benefits are numerous, but perhaps the most obvious is that walking improves your cardio fitness (aerobic capacity), which in turn lowers blood pressure, decreases levels of cholesterol and, according to a large-scale study of 72,000 women aged 40–65, substantially reduces risk of stroke and lowers breast cancer risk by up to 14 per cent. It can also decrease inflammation and blood-glucose levels, as well as improve depression scores. We personally like to use it to fuel creativity. While writing this book, we both clocked up hundreds of miles simply as a way to clear our heads, order our thoughts and get motivated – as well as procrastinate if we're being totally honest.

We're not the only ones who find a stroll good for generating ideas, though – researchers at Stanford University found walking can boost creativity by up to 60 per cent. The target often touted is 10,000 daily steps, but interestingly this has no real scientific basis and was actually chosen because it's a nice round number. By all means use it as a guide – either to aim for or to beat – but don't place too much emphasis on 10,000 steps and certainly don't invest in expensive wearables unless you have the money. Most smartphones have an in-built tracker that will give you a pretty good guide to the number you've racked up; as a general rule of thumb, an hour of moderate-paced walking equates to around 6,000 steps. While it's not essential to track your steps, it does mean you have a benchmark against which to note your progress, meaning you can push yourself by adding distance, pace, effort and incline.

Speaking of pace, anything that gets your heart pumping will deliver extra oxygen and nutrients to your muscles and your brain, so try increasing the rate and speed at which you walk and maybe add in some brisk arm movements. Crank it up a notch further to make more of a workout by incorporating steep hills, lunges, leg weights and interspersing short bursts of faster intervals. Running may get all the glory, but walking has definitely got legs when it comes to health and fitness gains.

There are several free walking apps available, including Pacer, Steps App, Map My Walk, Walkmeter, Footpath, Walk Fit, StepBet and Maipo.

Benefits of walking:

» Boosts mood by producing endorphins, which are the body's natural painkillers and mood elevators.
» Allows your mind to wander, which is useful if you're suffering from anxiety.
» A 12-minute walk can increase self-esteem and feelings of wellbeing.
» Walking for just 30 minutes can increase brain derived neurotrophic factor (BDNF) by 30 per cent. Low levels of BDNF have been linked with depression and dementia.
» Walking is classed as weight-bearing, so brings considerable benefits for bone health.
» It may reduce risk of respiratory conditions. In a study of 1,000 adults, those who walked 30–45 minutes a day had 43 fewer sick days and lower incidence of cold and flu than those who were sedentary.
» According to the mental health charity Mind, walking in nature improves mood, lowers stress, reduces anger and improves confidence – basically, it was made for perimenopausal women.

Using weights (resistance training)

Among its many important functions, oestrogen is anabolic – in other words, it helps to build muscle. As you've hopefully gathered by now, building muscle is one of the most important anti-ageing moves you can undertake. More muscle means increased physical strength, better bone health, higher stamina and, as a happy byproduct, you'll feel mentally fitter and more confident too. Nothing feels more kick-ass than deadlifting 60kg.

More muscle also means a higher resting metabolism, which can help with weight management (muscle burns around three times as many calories at rest as fat does).

Women often lose lean muscle as they age. Sarcopenia – the loss of muscle tone and mass – starts around your mid-30s, but many women only become aware of it as they hit their 40s. Women often say they no longer recognise their bodies, complaining they're softer, more rounded and less responsive to exercise.

There are a number of factors at play here. We lose about half a pound of lean muscle mass each year from around age 30 onwards. This depletion can be seen not just in muscle tone – you may notice your silhouette changes – but also in bone density, posture and physical stamina. To some degree, this is a natural part of ageing, but it's also down to declining hormones; oestrogen and testosterone are both crucial to muscle building. Many perimenopausal symptoms also affect our ability or motivation to exercise. Who the hell wants to work out after a night of disrupted sleep? Unwittingly, we also slow down as we get older.

In lieu of the muscle-building stimulus oestrogen and testosterone give us, we need to look for it elsewhere. This is where weights come in. Using an exercise programme incorporating weighted resistance training – dumbbells, gym equipment, resistance bands or your own body weight – two or three times a week (*every* week) can be nothing short of transformative. But you need to make it consistent and you need to constantly challenge yourself. Why? When you lift weights your body responds by upregulating muscle repair mechanisms to prevent what it perceives as damage. Over time this results in increased muscle mass (hypertrophy). To get tangible results, though, you need to slowly increase the intensity and load you're lifting. Trust us, your brain, heart, hormones and bones will thank you for it. Not just tomorrow, but in the years to come. By the way, we're not talking hour-long sessions here. Start with just 10 or 15 minutes and work up.

A quick-start guide to weights:

» YouTube is a stellar source of free workouts with body weight and dumbbell options. If you're new to weights, be sure to go at your pace and always warm up and stretch to cool down.
» Invest in some hand weights (between 1–5kg depending on your current strength levels), resistance bands or weighted arm/ankle straps. You can find lots online or use large bottles of water or a rucksack filled with books.
» Start low and slow and build up, but be consistent.
» Book in a few sessions with a personal trainer, who is experienced working with midlife women, to nail the basics and build confidence.
» Dismiss any fears about bulking up – you won't (ask any bodybuilder, it's just not that easy).

HIIT

There's a tendency for women to think they need to train harder and longer as they get older, all while eating less. The high levels of cortisol this can induce only serve to worsen perimenopause symptoms. So forget mammoth runs or hour-long spin sessions and look towards short, sharp bursts of getting the heart rate up. HIIT (high intensity interval training) offers a lot of bang for your buck and comes in a few forms, but essentially it involves a period of working hard, followed by a period of much lower intensity or complete rest. This is then repeated for a number of rounds or for a certain amount of time. That's not to say you should never run, and if you enjoy it and it's a staple part of your exercise regime then by all means stick with it, but if you're slogging it out on the treadmill or pounding pavements for long periods and finding your body composition isn't changing, then you might want to look at exercise that focuses on building muscle.

Typical functional body weight moves like burpees, squat jumps and press-ups feature heavily in HIIT classes, as can weighted exercises like overhead dumbbell presses and kettlebell swings. The beauty of HIIT is that if time is tight, you can squeeze an effective full-body workout into a mere 20 minutes. The reported benefits of HIIT stack up too: from fat burning to stamina to better sleep. No two ways about it, get HIIT right and you could become fitter than ever.

But there's a caveat. Due to its intensity, HIIT raises the heart rate, increases blood pressure and elevates your temperature – in effect, it puts you under acute (short-lived) stress and your body responds by producing antioxidants, regulating the fight-or-flight response and producing proteins and enzymes that mop up any damage. Many bodily maintenance and repair mechanisms are turned on by a HIIT workout and we see that in the 'after burn' effect – EPOC (exercise post-oxygen consumption), which increases your metabolism for a while after the workout has finished. All of this can be beneficial as long as your body is resilient enough to bounce back after being put under such pressure. However, if you're in the thick of perimenopause and struggling with overwhelm, insomnia and anxiety, undergoing super-intense forms of exercise may well make your symptoms worse; not only because it raises stress hormones, like cortisol, but because full recovery is thwarted as you're not sleeping. This puts you at extra risk of mood swings, fat storage around the middle and extreme fatigue. So while HIIT is beneficial, make sure you have your symptoms under control before you embark on a new programme and listen to your body. If it feels too much, stop, and always recover well (see below).

Yoga and Pilates

Many women advocate yoga and Pilates as a powerful mind-body tonic, so when the NICE guidelines listed them as bona fide perimenopause treatments it was a welcome stamp of approval. Both practices have their own merits and offer a number of techniques and approaches – from restorative hatha yoga to the core-challenging benefits of reformer bed Pilates.

The beauty of yoga and Pilates is that they're designed for everybody, but the key is to find a practice and instructor that is right for you. You might have to try out a few classes until you find 'the one', but stick with it as the rewards are plentiful.

For many perimenopausal women, the act of focusing on the breath, taking time to connect with the body and quietening a chattering mind are just some of the ways in which yoga and Pilates can help alleviate perimenopause symptoms. They both have their place when it comes to strengthening and sculpting the body too: as anyone who regularly sweats their way through an Ashtanga or a reformer bed session will attest. Then, of course, there are the benefits for muscle aches, digestion, tension, joint pain, pelvic floor health (libido), balance and blood pressure.

For the eye-rollers who think these practices are a bit woo woo, let's look at the science. A 2018 study found yoga to be as helpful as other exercise interventions when it came to reducing symptoms. Another study of 1,832 women linked yoga with a 'significant improvement in sleep'. On top of that, clinical trials suggest yoga can reduce inflammation, depression, anxiety and IBS. And Pilates has been shown to help with lower back pain, core strength and overall flexibility.

Think NEAT

NEAT (non-exercise activity thermogenesis) describes all the activity you do going about your normal day, including shopping, gardening, cleaning, popping to the post office, even running upstairs because you forgot something. It accounts for around 15 per cent of your total energy expenditure (much higher if you have a physically demanding job). So, while NEAT may be incidental, it has a significant bearing on your health and fitness levels. It's worth remembering even if you exercise for an hour a day five times a week, this only constitutes five hours or around three per cent of the whole week. Unsurprisingly, what you do for the remaining 165 hours is crucial. Incidentally, by increasing your levels of NEAT, you could be burning hundreds of calories daily, which adds up to thousands of additional calories weekly. Research shows people who increase NEAT gain less fat than people who aren't as active (see diagram below).

Sitting is not the new smoking

Sitting too much (research points to more than eight hours a day) is a problem, potentially leading to premature death

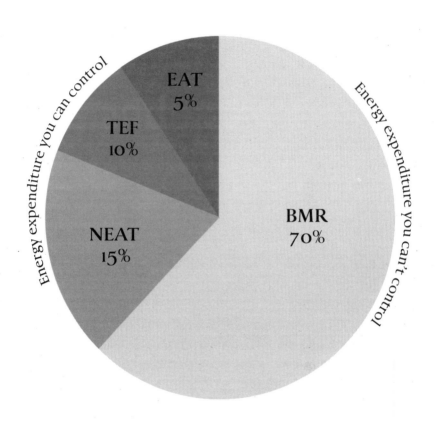

- **BMR** (*basal metabolic rate*): energy used for basic functions, e.g. breathing, blinking, heartbeat

- **NEAT** (*non-exercise activity thermogenesis*): non-intentional exercise, e.g. walking, gardening, housework

- **TEF** (*thermic effect of food*): energy used to digest food

- **EAT** (*exercise activity thermogenesis*): intentional exercise, e.g. workouts

APPROXIMATE DAILY ENERGY EXPENDITURE

and increasing some chronic diseases by 10–20 per cent, but let's be real, it doesn't compare to smoking – any claims that it does downplay the seriousness of smoking and are potentially misleading for the public. We do, however, need to be aware that sitting for long periods has the potential to affect the body's ability to regulate blood sugar, blood pressure and break down body fat.

According to the NHS, many adults in the UK spend around nine hours a day sitting. This includes watching TV, using a computer, reading, doing homework, travelling by car, bus or train, but doesn't include sleeping.

Here are a few ways to mitigate the effects of sitting, especially if you sit at a desk for long periods:

» Plan movement breaks every 30–45 minutes, even if it's just to stand and stretch.
» Buy a standing desk or an under-desk pedal machine, which is essentially the pedal unit you'd find on an exercise bike allowing you to pedal while you work.
» Walk and talk when you're on the phone; if you can do it outside, even better.
» Organise walking meetings (Steve Jobs swore by them).
» Have a glass of water next to you, and aim to get up and refill it every hour.

Over-exercising

An effective fitness regime relies as much on recovery as it does activity. We need to rest for muscle growth and repair, but also cell renewal, immune health and to regulate cortisol levels. Every woman is different, but for most perimenopausal clients we recommend working out no more than three or four days a week and we definitely advocate at least one of those sessions having more of a feel-good, restorative slant. Sessions that are too long create too much cortisol, which we know has a knock-on effect on insulin resistance, weight, sleep, anxiety and body-fat composition, so make sure you factor recovery days into your fitness schedule – they're as vital as the workouts themselves.

How much weekly exercise are we talking?
According to the NHS:

» At least 150 minutes of moderate aerobic activity (i.e. cycling, brisk walking). You should be out of breath but able to continue a conversation. Alternatively, 75 minutes of vigorous aerobic exercise (running, tennis, swimming).
» Plus at least two sessions of strength training that works all the major muscle groups: legs, hips, back, abdominals, chest, shoulders and arms.

The NHS website is a great place for ideas and how to get started https://www.nhs.uk/live-well/exercise

---

The bottom line

» All movement counts and it's never too late to start.
» Focus your attention on including some resistance training into your routine. Increased muscle mass is the name of the game during perimenopause.
» Yoga and Pilates can be useful for stretching, mindfulness and stress reduction.

» Think NEAT: all those little bursts of movement count – even fidgeting or mowing the lawn.

» Fill your days with exercise 'snacks'; you don't have to do all your exercise in one go. Break it up if that feels easier and less daunting.

CHAPTER 14

Supplements and Self-Care

If you have a tendency to eye-roll when someone mentions self-care, think again.

Lifestyle habits can have a strong influence on your perimenopause experience. Many women find they need to supplement their diet (and medical choices) with other, more holistic approaches to really optimise their health.

Anecdotally, and through our combined clinical experience, we've found many alternative approaches very helpful for the women we work with. This chapter outlines the options open to you. In it, we highlight the approaches that are useful and backed by science; we'll also discuss emerging therapies you might want to consider, but which haven't yet been substantiated by studies:

The power of placebo

The mind can be a powerful healing tool when given the chance, as illustrated by the placebo effect. In some clinical situations, a placebo (a fake treatment) has shown to be just as effective as scientific interventions. Why? We think there's lots of mechanisms at play but, as any health clinician knows, expectations play a role in a treatment's efficacy. In other words, the more you expect – and want – the treatment to work, the more likely you are to experience a positive outcome. The mind-body connection is incredibly powerful. But while placebos can affect how a person feels, they can't cure. A review that looked at more than 150 clinical trials involving placebos found they had no major clinical benefits, but did affect patient-reported outcomes, particularly when it came it came to nausea and pain.

Another theory is the act of taking a medication or carrying out a therapy has a positive healing effect, simply by dint of it being an act of self-care. Engaging in the tenets of healthy living – eating well, exercising, resting, hanging out with friends, getting quality sleep – provides many of the healing ingredients of the placebo effect. While these activities are positive interventions in their own right, focusing on them can enhance their benefits.

The attention and emotional support you give yourself isn't easily measured, but it leads to a feeling of wellbeing that can be invaluable during the transition through perimenopause. So, if you have a tendency to eye-roll when someone mentions self-care, you might want to think again.

Stress reduction

Long-term or chronic stress is one of the most overlooked factors in treating perimenopause. Throughout this book we've seen how sustained high levels of adrenaline and corti-sol negatively impact almost every system in the body: from the brain right down to the gut. Managing stress is one of the most critical parts of your perimenopause toolkit, and it's hard to think of a single symptom that isn't improved by calming your nervous system and reducing the impact on your adrenal health: brain fog, weight gain, IBS, acid reflux, thyroid dysfunction, hot flushes, palpitations, allergies, anxiety, irritability, headaches, insomnia and low libido are all made worse by stress.

There's nothing more enraging than someone else ramming their mindfulness regime down your throat, so think of the strategies below not as prescriptive, but as ideas to dip your toe in and try. But remember what we said above about self-care; perimenopause is absolutely the time to be taking this way of looking after yourself on board, however that might look for you.

Stimulate your vagus nerve

As well as connecting the brain and the gut, this balances out the fight-or-flight (stressed) state. Stimulating or 'massag-ing' the vagus nerve (see page 218) can trigger a relaxation response in the body. One of the quickest ways to do this is through deep breathing.

1. Breathe slowly, in through the nose and out through the mouth.
2. Breathe deeply into the belly as you inhale (think about expanding your rib cage. It can help to put your hands on either side of your rib cage and breathe into them).
3. Make your out-breath longer than your in-breath if you can. If you find it tricky, start by making them the same (a count of 4 in and 4 out) and then build up the out-breath to a count of 6 or 7.

Other activities to stimulate the vagus nerve include humming, laughing and singing. No wonder belting out karaoke tunes, in the company of others, makes you feel good. Chanting also has benefits and is just one of the reasons yoga sessions end with a collective 'ommmm'.

Movement

From walking in nature to short blasts on your cross-trainer or bike, exercise reduces stress and releases feel-good endorphins. Remember, in the name of balance and to minimise the effects of cortisol, for every high-octane workout, you need to counterbalance with proper rest and recovery. Over-training is very common in perimenopausal women and only serves to undermine your efforts.

Meditation

No longer reserved for yogis and monks, meditation is now an integral part of many discerning women's self-care regimes. In reality it's not always the easiest of practices, but meditation, mindfulness or just 'being in the moment' has been shown to have a calming effect on your nervous system and reduces the constant chatter and ruminating thoughts many perimenopausal women suffer from. It's not something you're likely to master in a day or even a month; it takes time and we think is best done either in the morning to set you up for the day ahead or at night to decompress and facilitate deep sleep, although there are no rules. If you want to give meditation a go, make sure your expectations are realistic; if you haven't done it before, quietening a noisy mind can be tough but persevere for at least a month. Start small, build up and enlist some help from an app – Headspace, Calm and Ten Percent Happier are three of the most popular ones.

Yoga

Yoga combines the benefits of breathing, mindfulness, movement and chanting. It is a lifesaver for many of the women we work with and is one of our most commonly 'prescribed' therapies. See page 241.

Cold therapy

Researchers believe exposure to cold activates vagus pathway neurons, triggers endorphins and improves immune health. There are many ways you can do it, including sea swimming, plunge pools and cryochambers, but a blast of cold water at the end of your shower for at least 30 seconds (building up to 5 minutes) is a good introduction. Research has shown that when cold therapy is carried out consistently, the body becomes more resilient and improves your response to stress in everyday life. Many perimenopausal women say its effects are transformative, making them feel sharper and brighter. It might also have a small fat burning effect.

Ellie's story

During perimenopause a series of unforeseen personal traumas hit me – one after another – and my inner world started to crumble. Then the anxiety struck. I wasn't in a good place, but I felt paralysed and unable to do anything about it. I wanted out.

I started taking antidepressants, but they made me feel incredibly sick so I had to come off them. I'd heard of cold-water swimming helping with depression and anxiety. I didn't really believe it, but I felt desperate, so I decided to go with it.

At first it was hard, it takes time to control your breathing and not give in to the shock of the temperature, but it was so transformative I couldn't believe it wasn't on prescription. The immersion in water is an immediate meditation. Your brain can think of nothing other than the sensations in your body. The water takes everything: all the troubles, anxiety, worry, sadness, grief; it takes it all and gives you back yourself. Little by little I was pieced back together again by the sea. It sounds crazy but the sea saved my life.

Supplements

In an ideal world we'd get all the vitamins and minerals we need from food. In reality, life is busy. Stress, work, poor sleep, alcohol, gut health issues and skipped meals all increase the likelihood we fall short on nutrients that could help optimise our perimenopause experience. Both of us regularly speak to women who are taking reams – we're talking carrier bags full – of pills and potions. It's not hard to see why; women who haven't been able to get the help they so desperately need – who aren't understood or properly listened to – often end up taking their health into their own hands and Dr Google can lead them down a worm hole that suggests they need more than they do. Not only are many of the supplements marketed at perimenopausal women expensive and often unnecessary, they have the potential to do harm.

There's a tendency towards thinking 'natural' is harmless, when in fact many of the remedies you can buy online and in-store are incredibly potent. Herbs, in particular, can interact with prescription medicines – don't forget some types of chemotherapy have plant derivative ingredients that are far from harmless – and certain vitamins in high doses can be lethal. Vitamin A, for example, has been shown to increase a smoker's risk of getting lung cancer, too much

B6 can cause irreparable nerve damage, calcium supplements have been linked to kidney stones and high doses of selenium are toxic and lead to hair loss. Our advice: know what you're taking; don't just pop pills and tinctures willy-nilly. The website drugs.com is a good place to check for minor interactions between medications and food/supplements, and if you're starting any new regime and are taking existing medication, make sure to let your doctor know. Below is a conservative list of some of the recommended supplements we most commonly use in clinic. That doesn't mean they're right for you. It's impossible – not to mention unprofessional – to give out blanket advice on supplements. In order to give a well-rounded protocol, a practitioner needs to consider any existing medication and potentially contra-indicating supplements you're taking. We'd also need to have a detailed overview of your health record to date, so it's vital that you speak to a qualified healthcare practitioner before using any kind of supplements, especially if you're taking a blood thinner like Warfarin, anti-depressants, HRT or blood pressure medication.

If you think you'd benefit from more individualised support, book in with a registered nutritionist or other specialist in this field.

Magnesium

Magnesium is used in over 600 bodily reactions, from relaxing muscles and regulating blood-sugar levels, to producing energy. It calms the nervous system and supports the adrenal glands, so plays an important role in dealing with stress. Interestingly, magnesium works in harmony with serotonin (see page 218) and melatonin (see page 139) so it's a pretty big deal.

Magnesium is widely available from food (see page 184), but according to the World Health Organization, up to 75 per cent of the population are possibly deficient. This can lead to tiredness, weakness, palpitations, cramps and eye twitches. Alcohol and stress use up your body's magnesium stores. Magnesium deficiency is linked with insulin resistance so often seen in those with Type 2 diabetes, and if you have an inflammatory bowel disorder like Crohn's, you might well lose magnesium through diarrhoea. For women in perimenopause who have anxiety, restless legs, aching muscles, sleep issues, migraines and high blood pressure, magnesium may be very helpful. The upper limit for magnesium supplements is 300–400mg a day and there are lots of different types: magnesium glycinate is good for calming, magnesium malate helps with muscle relaxation, magnesium threonate for brain function, magnesium taurate aids blood-sugar control and magnesium citrate is good for constipation. If you want to try one but aren't sure which is best, the most easily absorbed all-rounder is magnesium glycinate. As well as capsules and powders, you can buy magnesium in a spray form for restless legs and muscle aches, or dissolve two big handfuls of Epsom salts in a warm bath and soak for 20 minutes as magnesium can be absorbed through the skin.

Omega 3

Omega 3 has an anti-inflammatory effect on the body and makes up the outer membrane of every cell in your body, helping cells to signal to each other and also sealing in hydration. The best source of Omega 3 is to eat oily fish (see page 172), but for vegans and vegetarians – or those who dislike the taste or smell – this isn't possible. An Omega 3 supplement can make up the deficit and also works to balance out high levels of Omega 6 (found in processed foods like crisps and cooking oils such as sunflower oil), which can be inflammatory and which many of us over-consume.

Low levels of Omega 3 can show up as dry, scaly skin, hair loss, keratosis pilaris (small bumps on the back of your arms) and psoriasis. Research suggests Omega 3 might be helpful for depression; anxiety; eye, heart and brain health; rheumatoid arthritis and asthma, and may even help reduce the inflammation associated with Alzheimer's. There's no agreed dose when it comes to supplementing, although for therapeutic amounts look for around 500mg EPA and 500 DPA on the label and make sure the brand offers a 'high purity' assurance. Vegans and non-fish eaters should opt for an algae oil.

B vitamins

All eight B vitamins (B1, B2, B3, B5, B6, B7, B9, B12) play a unique role in the body, but collectively they work to support energy levels and mental health. Deficiencies in any one of them can lead to serious problems: low B12 can mimic the symptoms of dementia, sub-optimal B6 can impact progesterone production and, if you don't have sufficient B9, you may experience palpitations and increase your risk of heart disease. The consensus is unanimous: don't underestimate the importance of B vitamins during perimenopause. They're also water-soluble, meaning they're not stored in the body, so they need to be consumed regularly.

You can find B vitamins in many foods including liver, seafood, chicken, eggs, lentils, leafy greens, fortified foods (like plant milks and nutritional yeast) and seeds. Annoyingly, B vitamins are lost from foods when we cook them – this is particularly true of over-boiled vegetables, which is why steaming is always best (see page 279). The body uses lots of B vitamins to metabolise alcohol and deal with stress. Be aware that B2 makes your wee neon yellow, so don't be alarmed.

Lastly, it's important to note B12 is only found in animal products. The Vegan Society recommends non-meat eaters take a 10mcg B12 supplement daily or 2000mcg weekly.

Women over the age of 50 and anyone taking the prescription drug, Metformin, are also recommended to supplement as B12 absorption is impacted in both scenarios.

Vitamin D

We need vitamin D for strong bones (it works in harmony with calcium), to support our immune system and combat low mood and anxiety. Low levels are also thought to play a part in insulin resistance (see page 162). Vitamin D is found in pretty paltry amounts in food, so the most efficient way to get it is by exposing your skin to sunlight – just 20 minutes a day is thought to be enough, though this can be hard in the northern hemisphere, especially in winter months. Sunscreen use, cancer risk, the British climate, time spent indoors and religious clothing that covers the skin mean many of us simply aren't getting enough vitamin D.

Public Health England recommends all adults in the UK supplement with at least 10mcg (400IU) of vitamin D when sun is at its lowest (from October to March). Women with darker skin tones or gut issues may well need a higher dose of up to 25mcg (1000IU) or possibly more. If in doubt, your doctor can test your levels, which we would strongly advise, as low vitamin D can mimic early-stage perimenopause symptoms (optimal levels are 70–80nmol/L). Vitamin D works best alongside vitamin K2, which deposits calcium into the bone and helps prevent fractures. Look for a supplement that combines the active forms of both: D3 + K2. There are many on the market, including sprays which offer a convenient option and which are best to take with a meal that contains fat.

Inositol

There is some evidence for supplementing with myo-inositol (a naturally occurring substance in the body that's similar to sugar) to improve insulin sensitivity in metabolic disorders such as PCOS, gestational diabetes and metabolic syndrome, which can occur in perimenopause. A number of recent studies have found myo-inositol helps to increase the body's ability to tolerate glucose. It also improves hormonal balance, lowers excess testosterone (often the cause of acne in PCOS) and supports ovulation. Some studies point to it supporting reductions in anxiety symptoms too. Most of the trials to date have used a daily dose of 2–4g, but talk to a registered nutrition professional to work out the right dosage for you.

Vegan diet support

The following nutrients all need to be considered when on a vegan diet as there is a risk of deficiencies: B12, zinc, iron, iodine, choline, taurine, vitamin D, vitamin A, vitamin K2 and Omega 3 fatty acids. Not all are recommended in a supplement form, i.e. iodine needs to be managed very carefully to avoid over-stimulating the thyroid. To ensure you're optimising your diet – and doing it as safely as possible – it's advisable to get guidance from a nutritionist.

Multivitamins

If your diet is severely lacking and you don't have the means or time to address it, then a certain school of thought says it might be worth taking a basic multivitamin, almost as an insurance policy. Most multivitamins have such a wide margin of safety, even when you're combining them with fortified foods, they're likely to be safe. However, if you're taking a multivitamin on top of other vitamins and minerals, you may well be exceeding the recommended daily intake.

When it comes to vitamins as a whole, it's worth considering that a large review of 27 vitamin trials – consisting of over 400,000 people – concluded people who took vita-mins were not necessarily healthier, did not live longer or have fewer cases of chronic disease compared to non-pill poppers. Our advice is to always work on getting the foun-dations of good nutrition in place first (see Chapter 10), before you start thinking about adding supplements into the mix.

The non-HRT options

Many women look to herbal remedies or supplements because they're worried about the risks or aren't sure of the benefits of Hormone Replacement Therapy (HRT). They argue that they want a more 'natural' approach – after all menopause is a natural event, so why medicalise it with drugs? Whatever you decide – and it is of course your choice – first ensure you have the facts to hand. Do you not want to take HRT because of the bad press it has received in the past? Do you have concerns over its safety? We've covered these issues in Chapter 4, so if you need to, go back and refresh your memory. It's crucial that you talk to some-one about *your* situation and *your* medical history. Nobody else's. All too often we come across women who are deny-ing themselves a form of treatment without full evidence and understanding.

That said, we totally understand that taking HRT (or not) is a personal choice and for a group of women who've had breast cancer or are at a high risk of breast cancer, in particular, then it's not automatically a valid option. We're here to look at all the different options to help you make your decision. If you have made an active choice to not take HRT, there are still several options open to you, including over-the-counter supplements and pharmacological treat-ments your doctor can prescribe to ease your symptoms.

Other prescription medications

If you're experiencing hot flushes and night sweats, what we call vasomotor symptoms, there is a group of antidepressants called SSRIs (selective serotonin reuptake inhibitors) and SSNRIs (selective serotonin and noradrenaline reuptake inhibitors) that are typically used to treat depression and anxiety and can ease symptoms of fatigue, anxiety and insomnia. Venlafaxine is often the first choice for breast cancer survivors. Side-effects include a dry mouth, nausea, constipation and they can lower libido or make it more difficult to orgasm. Tibolone is similar to taking combined HRT, but can have side-effects. If you're unsure, your doctor can talk you through the type of medication that's right for you.

You may have heard of gabapentin, a drug typically used for chronic pain that can also help reduce hot flushes and sweats. Bear in mind it can cause drowsiness in the daytime, so needs to be started at a low dose and increased slowly. Clonidine is a drug that was initially used for lowering blood pressure and is now the first non-hormonal drug in the UK to be licensed for hot flushes.

Herbal remedies

When it comes to herbs (and supplements too) there tends to be a scattergun approach, partly due to the fact that there aren't many robust studies. If you want to go down the herbal route, we strongly suggest you speak to a registered herbalist through the National Institute of Medical Herbalists at www.nimh.org.uk. NICE guidelines recommend that you look for the THR (Traditional Herbal Registration) mark on the label. Inform your doctor as some herbal remedies can interfere with prescription medications.

These are the herbs most commonly used to help alleviate perimenopause symptoms.

Herb	Symptom
Black cohosh	Vasomotor symptoms such as night sweats and hot flushes, low mood (not recommended for anyone with liver problems).
St John's Wort	Mild depression, anxiety, insomnia and mood swings. Can be used by women with a history or at high risk of breast cancer (not to be taken alongside Tamoxifen).
Red clover	Hot flushes (used with caution in women with oestrogen-sensitive cancers, endometriosis or fibroids because of its oestrogen-mimicking properties.
Ashwagandha	Poor sleep, anxiety, stress.
Agnus castus (also known as vitex, chasteberry or chaste-tree)	PMS, irritability, low mood, irregular periods.
Maca	Hot flushes, night sweats, insomnia, libido, anxiety.
Sage	Hot flushes.
Gingko biloba	Memory and brain function, low libido.
Rhodiola	Fatigue, low mood, stress.
Holy basil	Stress, memory, cognitive function.
Lemon balm	Stress, anxiety, memory, low mood, poor sleep.

Complementary therapies

Acupuncture: this involves inserting very fine needles into specific sites in the body for therapeutic or preventative purposes. It is used in many NHS GP practices these days, as well as in most pain clinics and hospices in the UK. Robust evidence is lacking when it comes to acupuncture's efficacy for perimenopause, but anecdotally many women find it helps with a number of hormone and mood-related symptoms, including hot flushes, pain, PMS and even burning mouth syndrome. A small study in the *British Medical Journal* prompted researchers to conclude acupuncture provides 'a realistic' treatment option for women who are unable to or don't want to use HRT. Our opinion is acupuncture is safe and can be restorative (choose a practitioner who specialises in women's health), so if it's something you can afford, it can be a worthwhile addition to your self-care arsenal. However, if you've tried it for 3–4 sessions and haven't felt any benefits, it's probably best to save your money.

Cognitive Behavioural Therapy (CBT): is a therapeutic intervention that challenges unhelpful thoughts, feelings and behaviours. It is most commonly used to develop coping strategies for dealing with symptoms such as anxiety and depression. Many women find CBT a helpful and safe way to reduce the frequency and duration of hot flushes. This is largely because hot flushes are often triggered – and made more intense – by stress. The British Menopause Society recommends CBT for a number of perimenopause symptoms, including sleep, and NICE flags it as a useful treatment for depression, poor self-esteem and low mood.

CBD oil (Cannabidiol): this is made from phytocannabinoids – active compounds produced by cannabis plants – but doesn't contain THC (tetrahydrocannabinol), the psychoactive part that makes you high. It is, therefore, completely legal in the UK and not addictive. Phytocannabinoids work by interacting with receptors in the body's endocannabinoid system that support balance and wellness. There's some promising evidence emerging (though more controlled clinical studies on large sample sizes are needed before we can determine dosages and outcomes) for CBD oil's benefits for pain, insomnia, inflammation, anxiety and sleep, which in turn can help gut health issues, hot flushes, night sweats, fatigue and maybe even migraines. Bear in mind, though, while the CBD industry is expanding fast, it's currently a very poorly regulated area and CBD products aren't cheap, so ask questions about the purity, dosages and strengths before you buy. Any respectable brand will be able to tell you everything you need to know and should have carried out independent, third-party testing, known as COA (certificate of analysis). We suggest looking for a broad spectrum oil (i.e. whole plant extract, not an isolate) that's made from hemp, starting with a low dose and building up. The Food Standards Agency recommend a maximum daily dose of 70mg. Everyone responds to CBD differently and we've heard too many stories about women going hell for leather and then feeling wired as a result, which wasn't their desired outcome.

The bottom line

»   The placebo effect is real (and can be very effective).
»   Supplements should never replace a healthy lifestyle, balanced diet, exercise and good sleep.
»   Everyone in the UK should take at least 10mcg (possibly up to 25mcg) of vitamin D between October and March.
»   If you have a medical condition or take any medications, consult with your healthcare provider before embarking on any course of supplements.

» If you want to try herbal medicines, ideally consult with a registered herbalist. If that's not possible and you're buying herbal tinctures off the shelf, look for the THR registration stamp on the label.

» Acupuncture and CBT can be useful additions to your perimenopause toolkit.

» CBD oil is becoming popular among perimenopausal women to help with sleep and anxiety. Always check for purity before buying – ask the company for clarification if you're unsure.

CHAPTER 15

47 Ways to Lose Fat that Don't Involve Calorie Counting

You're aiming for consistency, not perfection.

Perimenopausal women will often say their body appeared to thicken and grow soft overnight. Their loudest lament is that they feel their weight is out of their control. Most feel guilty for wanting to address it, like they're bad feminists; but there's two things to consider here. Firstly, perimenopause-induced weight gain doesn't happen overnight; it often starts in your 30s. Secondly, it's perfectly ok to want to do something about it; your body, your choice. In this chapter we'll look at why weight gain is such a common complaint, the many reasons it happens and what can be done about it, if indeed you want to do something at all. If weight management isn't relevant, doesn't appeal or is triggering, skip this chapter altogether. Eating disorders are on the rise among midlife women, so if you need help or more information, the BEAT website (see page 299) is a good place to start.

Statistics report we put on an average of half to one kilo a year from our mid-30s. Over the course of ten years, that can mean a couple of extra dress sizes. It creeps up slowly, almost imperceptibly, until one day you wake up and, boom, there it is. The added surprise is it all seems to accumulate around your mid-section. Why? Your basal metabolic rate (BMR) is the energy you need to simply stay alive: to breathe, to keep your heart beating, to circulate blood. As you age it slows down, meaning you need a lower energy intake in your 40s than you did in your 20s.

In addition, many of us unwittingly become more sedentary during midlife; hormonal fluctuations mean we're often fatigued and, in turn, our desire to exercise becomes blunted. Not to mention the fact that fat cells produce small amounts of oestrogen, which of course your body wants to hang on to at all costs. Add stress into the mix, which encourages fat to be laid down around the middle, some genetics, plus loss of insulin sensitivity (see page 162), and you have the perfect storm for weight gain.

Weight gain in itself isn't necessarily a health issue. The health at every size (HAES) movement is re-educating commonly held fat-phobic perceptions – particularly in the medical world – that women in larger bodies can be fit, strong and healthy, and rightly so. But for women who are living with obesity and who aren't active, there are long-term health associations that are hard to ignore: Type 2 diabetes, heart disease, joint pain, dementia and breast cancer. Around sixty per cent of British women are over-weight or obese, and the biggest proportion is among those aged 45–54. This chapter is not about fat-shaming or about aesthetics; it's about overall health and improving quality of life, life expectancy and reducing the severity of your symptoms.

Weight loss should be so easy: eat fewer calories, move more. So why doesn't it work for most women? Maybe because trying to lose weight by focusing on food is like trying to quit drinking by focusing on alcohol. In clinic, the best results occur when women look at their eating habits and behaviours, rather than focusing on calories. Unsurprisingly, too, there isn't a one-size-fits-all solution. Weight loss is multi-layered at any time of life, but it's extra nuanced during perimenopause. Your genetics and microbiome (the good bacteria that live in your gut) play a part, so does your environment, your job, your family and your socio-economic background. Like we said, it's complex.

Your toolbox

Personalised nutrition is the way forward, but in the absence of lengthy consultations and in-depth testing, here is a tool-box of ideas that you can put in place. Some you may have tried, some might be new. Others you might be re-visiting for a third, fourth or fifth time because, let's face it, fat loss is never linear. It takes time and patience, and a bit of trial and error.

Go through the list and highlight any that immediately jump out at you that seem practical and fit in around your job, family and lifestyle. They might need a little tweak here and there and if at first you don't succeed, stop, reflect, take on board what you've learnt, and start over the following day.

Prep your breakfast

Whatever time you decide to have breakfast, make sure your first meal of the day has plenty of protein, fibre and some healthy fats (remember the Key 3 from page 182) to set up nice steady blood-sugar levels for the day.

Go against the graze

Most people function better with 2–3 balanced, satiating meals, rather than grazing all day. If you're eating frequently, your body never gets to the point where it's breaking into its fat stores. The key is to make your breakfast mighty, so it can keep you going for a few hours until it's time to eat again.

Think fat loss, not weight loss

Water retention, where you are in your menstrual cycle, fluctuating hormones and whether or not you've been to the toilet can all impact weight. Fat loss is a better goal. Judge progress by how your clothes feel or by progress photos, rather than the scales.

Make protein a priority

Protein (see page 169) is the most satiating macro (very hard to overeat), helps preserve muscle mass and keeps metabolism revved. Before you make each meal, ask yourself where your protein source is.

Lean on iodine

We need iodine to keep our thyroid functioning optimally and many of us are deficient. Low thyroid activity can mean weight gain, lethargy and sluggish digestion. You'll find iodine in prawns, seaweed and dairy, or try swapping your regular salt for iodised salt.

Eat less stuff from packets

The more you prep your own meals, the more control you have over what goes in them. Processed foods often contain far more sugar, fat and salt than you'd ever use at home.

Add in, don't take away

Think about what you can include, rather than remove from your diet. Crowd out the unhealthier food in your life with a glut of better, more health-giving options like fresh vegetables and salads.

Pinpoint your hunger window

Not hungry when you wake up? Push your first meal back to later in the day. If you wake up starving but you're not hungry at lunch, eat a big breakfast and skip lunch. Eating intuitively can help reduce your intake without counting calories.

Track your progress

Buy a cheap paper calendar that displays the entire year on one page. Mark each day that you manage to stick to your goal with a big red cross. Trying to create a continuous line of crosses – no gaps – can be very motivating.

Sort out your snacks

Plan and prep healthy snacks so that you have them to hand: examples are boiled eggs, celery and nut butter, chopped vegetables and hummus, roasted chickpeas.

Curb the cravings

When cravings crop up, stop and question if they're down to genuine hunger or boredom, loneliness, stress, habit, etc. Do you notice any patterns? Does eating the food you crave address the feeling? If it doesn't, make a list of alternative activities that you could do: maybe go for a walk, call a friend, put your favourite tune on loudly and dance, make a cup of tea, read a book, listen to a podcast or write in your journal.

Marion's story

I'm a social care worker in a deprived borough of London. My job is stressful, my hours are long and I rely on food for comfort, not least to block out troubling thoughts, particularly if I'm dealing with a traumatic case.

Perimenopause hit me hard: my weight sky-rocketed, I couldn't sleep, I started having panic attacks and my relationship with my wife was in free-fall. My coping mechanism was to eat my way through it, but at a Well Woman check my doctor flagged up my high blood pressure and spiralling weight and suggested my heart health wouldn't be able to cope much longer. It was the kick up the bum I needed.

The first thing to go was the weekday drinking, which surprisingly quickly helped my sleep and my state of mind. I've always been reluctant when it comes to fitness, but when I started sleeping better I felt I had the energy to exercise. And the more exercise I did, the more I realised I loved how it made me feel. The natural progression was then to take a good long look at my diet. It's now been 18 months and I'm feeling (and looking) a lot lighter.

My biggest realisation is that health is a journey. Nothing happens overnight, so you have to enjoy – and to a degree trust – the process, particularly when it doesn't feel like anything much is changing. It's about consistency, not perfection.

Volume of veg

Vegetables fill you up, stretch your stomach and turn off the hunger hormone, ghrelin. Go large. Roast big trays of them, make soups, shoehorn them into sandwiches and salads, blend them into sauces, turn them into noodles (you can buy small handheld spiralisers for under a tenner), make courgette lasagne, add them to casseroles, stuff them into peppers and try cauliflower rice.

Trick your brain

The bigger the plate you're eating from, the more likely you are to fill it. Eating from a smaller plate gives you the illusion that your meal is larger than it is.

Fill your boots with greens

Have some greens at each meal, including breakfast, when you can. They're low in energy but big on flavour and good-ness. Keep a bag of mixed leaves in the fridge and add them wherever you can to sandwiches, scrambled eggs/tofu, smoothies, curries, stews or dahl.

Quench your appetite

Ghrelin (your hunger hormone) is released when your stom-ach is empty. Water fills you up and can turn ghrelin off temporarily. Make sure you're getting around 2 litres a day (you might need more if you're exercising).

Have you tried IF?

Intermittent fasting (IF) is by no means a fast track to fat loss, but some women find it very helpful, particularly if they're big late-night snackers. There are many ways to go about it, but the easiest is what's known as time-restricted eating. Simply choose an eating window – try 7am to 7pm – and make sure you only eat within that timeframe. You could then try extending it to 10am–8pm and then maybe even 12pm–8pm. Be aware, though, that if your perimenopause symptoms have the better of you right now – you're exhausted, low, sleeping badly – intermittent fasting is not a sensible approach. You have to trust us on this – it's an added stress you simply do not need and will more than likely backfire. It is also not advisable if you have thyroid issues or a history of disordered eating.

Stomach hungry or mouth hungry?

Stomach hungry is when your belly is rumbling – it's been a few hours since your last meal and you feel empty. Mouth hunger is just about fancying something to eat. Be aware of the difference.

Put a full stop at the end of a meal

Don't be afraid to have something sweet if it means you're going to be yearning for it all day/night otherwise. Try a Medjool date with a teaspoon of nut butter, a few squares of dark chocolate or a small chia pudding.

What's your motivation?

Visualise your goal (cut pictures out) or make it digital (Pinterest). It doesn't have to be aesthetic, it can be a feeling, a mood, an emotion, an action. This isn't woo woo; it's a technique used by many top sports stars. Spend five minutes looking at your vision board every day and immersing yourself in the pictures.

It's a numbers game

Try to focus your efforts on positive numbers – kilos of weight lifted in the gym, steps walked, number of vegetables you've eaten – rather than numbers on scales.

Deprivation leads to desire

Omitting things entirely – no chocolate, no carbs, no caffeine – isn't just difficult, it can make you obsess over that restricted item and eventually over-consume. Allow some room to stray in your new regime: 80:20 is a good guide.

Get handy

To help with portion control, think a palm-sized portion of protein, a small fist of carbs, a thumb of healthy fats (and as many vegetables as possible).

Invest in a CGM (continuous glucose monitor).

Low blood sugar is one of the principle drivers of hunger and can make you anxious, stressed, panicky and desperate for a quick sugar fix. Monitoring your levels using a CGM can be a really useful insight and help you maintain equilibrium (see box).

Continuous glucose monitors (CGM)

Blood glucose monitors, which can be bought at pharmacies and online, are small, flat sensors you attach to your arm (painlessly). Originally created for people with various forms of diabetes, their relevance is applicable to anyone looking to better understand their blood glucose fluctuations. They link to an app that tracks your blood-glucose levels on a graph. CGMs take the guesswork out of how the food you eat is affecting your blood glucose levels. For best results, work alongside a nutritionist who can analyse your results and suggest dietary adaptations. Emma regularly uses Freestyle Libre in her clinic – each sensor lasts two weeks and costs around £50–£70.

Strength in numbers

Find a local group, a Facebook community or just a friend who is aiming for the same end goal as you. It will help you stay accountable, give you a reason to show up each day and also support you when you start to waiver.

Mindful eating

Taking time to savour your meals can help manage overeating. Make sure you're seated rather than eating on the go, chew each bite really well and put your cutlery down between mouthfuls. Remove any distractions, such as your phone or laptop, and turn off the TV during mealtimes.

Address your stress

Stress is one of the biggest obstacles to fat loss as it puts your body in survival mode (see box). If you're time poor, try a 5-minute guided mindfulness meditation or if that's not your thing, just breathe (see page 249): deep belly breathing helps your parasympathetic 'calm' state kick in.

Stress, exercise and an inability to lose fat

Stress – from over-exercising, working long hours, chronic inflammation, insufficient sleep – raises cortisol and puts your body into survival mode.

This means it releases stored glucose from your muscles and liver into the bloodstream, ready for fight or flight. Cortisol increases carb cravings as it wants your body to have plenty of glucose to be able to flee from the stressful situation it thinks is imminent. Cortisol also reduces your thyroid's effectiveness, which in turn lowers your metabolism. On top of all this, when under stress, your body wants to conserve energy at all costs, as an insurance policy, so it holds on to fat stores for dear life. Some women respond to this inability to lose fat by working out harder than ever, which simply ups cortisol further and compounds the issue even more.

Stress can show up in many guises: feeling overwhelmed, lonely, tearful, joyless, anxious and unable to see the point of life. It might manifest as fast breathing, muscle tension, headaches, low libido, sleep problems, constipation and diarrhoea or panic attacks. There are many ways to manage stress – from meditation to cold-water swimming – but the most important thing is to recognise it and address it. Don't ignore stress and hope it'll go away. Start today by saying 'no' to stuff you don't want to or can't do. It's time to make your needs – and your health – a priority.

Keep it on the low low

When you're choosing your carbs, think low glycemic load options (i.e. slow energy release): brown basmati rice, oats, green leafy vegetables, berries, cherries, plums, kiwis, apples, pears.

Lose fat, not sleep?

Being tired can make you eat more. Studies show a poor night's sleep can result in eating an extra 200–400 calories of snacks the next day as cravings for salty, sweet and high-sugar foods increase by 30–40 per cent. To get your sleep on track, see Chapter 8.

Emergency recipe

Learn one failsafe, quick, easy, healthy recipe from staples that you always have in your cupboard; something you can knock up when you're tired, hungry, time poor or haven't been to the shops.

Inspect your gadgets

Would your healthy eating efforts be made easier by investing in an appliance? NutriBullets are great for making smoothies, dressings and dips and a stick blender blasts through soups. Digital scales can help with portion control. A slow cooker is a godsend if you want to come home to a ready-cooked, hot meal.

Get NEAT

Non exercise thermogenesis activity (NEAT) is all the movement you do that's not planned exercise and it can make or break a fat-loss plan. Up your step count, mow the lawn, take the stairs instead of the lift, walk up escalators; it all counts. Just. Keep. Moving.

Set yourself up for success

Make your new healthy habits as easy to execute as possible. Get your yoga mat out the night before, put your dumbbells somewhere obvious, make a protein smoothie and have it waiting in the fridge, have your gym gear next to your bed, cue your YouTube workout, compile a running playlist.

Remove temptation

Don't keep hyper-palatable, energy-dense food in the house. If you have to have it (because … kids) keep in an opaque jar and keep that jar out of sight.

Go slow and steady

You can't force fat loss, and the more aggressively you try, the harder it is to stick to. Make your goals achievable and stay realistic: 0.5–1kg total body weight loss a week is a manageable target for most.

Get real with your expectations

When dreams and reality are at odds, you dramatically reduce your chances of success. In one study, half the participants with unrealistic expectations dropped out within a year of starting their healthy eating plan.

Don't over-exercise

Hammering your body into submission doesn't help fat loss in perimenopause. Too much exercise causes high cortisol, which can encourage your body to store fat around the middle. Exercise regularly and make it challenging, but make sure you build in recovery time.

Pasta lovers

Swap white pasta for high-protein alternatives, like pea or edamame pasta, available from health-food shops or online. It provides slower-release energy, is more filling and adds fibre.

Testosterone boost

Testosterone gel can help with increased muscle mass (and therefore reduced fat loss) and the motivation needed to exercise. Talk to your doctor as it can be prescribed off-label, alongside HRT, for women during perimenopause.

Mindset maintenance

Need some tips on goal-setting and making new habits stick? Here's your 10-step guide:

1. Set SMART goals: Specific, Measurable, Attainable, Relevant, Timed.
2. Know your what, why and how. What is your goal? Why do you want it? How will it make a difference to your life? When faced with a situation that might derail your healthy habits plan, ask yourself the question: 'How is this helping my goal?' If the answer is 'it's not', try to swerve it.
3. Think long-term: it's crucial you trust – and enjoy – the process.
4. Visualise where you'll be in three months if you keep making changes each week.
5. Start to identify as this new, slightly tweaked version of yourself. It's important you embrace the actions and mindset required to achieve your goal.
6. List your actions and steps, so you know what your plan looks like. Write them out, refer back to them frequently and amend and update them as you progress.
7. Tag your new habit(s) on to something that's already part of your routine, i.e. squats while brushing your teeth (habit stacking) or getting your breakfast ingredients together while waiting for the kettle to boil.
8. Think of your goal as a process, rather than fixating on the end result: every day you get stronger/faster/more resilient/more energised.

9. Consider obstacles that might crop up or have scuppered plans when you've tried to adopt new healthy behaviours in the past. Write them down. Now come up with solutions to overcome them.

10. Recognise your successes along the way. Celebrate the small wins as they happen. Each one is worth shouting about and is another step closer to your end goal.

Cut the cardio

Resistance/strength training is the way forward when it comes to perimenopausal fat loss (see page 238): it helps to increase lean muscle mass, which raises metabolic rate, increases insulin sensitivity, burns fat and doesn't increase ghrelin as much as cardio. That doesn't mean you can't run or do a spin class; just keep it short (30 mins) and don't make it your main form of exercise.

Plan ahead

Meal plans can help take the surprise element out of eating and set you up for success. Spend half an hour on a Sunday batch-cooking a few meals and plotting out roughly how your week of eating is going to look.

Have a booze break

Drinking alcohol is one of the biggest saboteurs of healthy eating. It's high in energy, increases your hunger and doesn't help you make good food choices. Have some delicious, alcohol-free options lined up: flavoured sugar-free kombucha (see page 223) is good and has gut benefits too.

Cooking hacks

» Watch a short knife skills tutorial on YouTube (try 'Jamie Oliver on Knife Skills'). It will save you heaps of time when it comes to prepping vegetables.

» Keep a jar of mixed seeds handy to add to soups, stir-fries and salads.

» Build your spice collection over time.

» If you don't have a steamer, fill a saucepan with an inch of boiling water on the hob on a medium heat. Place the veg inside, pop on a lid and leave for 10 minutes or so.

» Keep old jars and bottles or invest in some kilner jars for batch-prepping breakfasts like chia pudding and overnight oats and to store leftovers.

» Always shake your plant milk before using as the added calcium settles on the bottom.

» Keep some pre-cooked pouches of grains in the cupboard. Merchant Gourmet do good ones – including puy lentils, quinoa, cous cous, freekeh – that don't have any additives, stabilisers or preservatives.

Don't eat like an influencer

Social media stars go all out to make their food get likes. There's no way they eat a smoothie bowl that big all to themselves, or that packed with peanut butter, tahini, dark chocolate and cacao nibs.

Have a cup of Joe

Drinking caffeine before a workout can enhance performance, mood, motivation and energy. But avoid if you're
sensitive to it, especially on an empty stomach as it can
elevate cortisol and blood glucose.

Take it easy

Do whatever it takes to make eating well easier: buy chopped
garlic, sliced onions, pre-cooked meat and fish (smoked
salmon, mackerel fillets, grilled chicken), ready-to-cook
stir-fry veg, frozen chopped mixed vegetables, pouches of
rice, grains and lentils. If you can afford it, go one step further
and order recipe kits from companies like Mindful Chef or
Gousto.

Stop scrolling

Got no time to batch cook/walk/do yoga, but spend hours
on Instagram? Maybe it's time to re-think your phone habits.

Be mindful of the extras

All the little bites and nibbles and slurps add up. Finishing
off the kids' leftovers is a common one.

Keep a food diary

We all – even nutritionists – tend to underestimate how
much we eat in a day. Tracking it takes the guesswork out,
makes you more aware of what you're consuming and helps
highlight the triggers or times of day when eating goes awry.
You don't need to do this for weeks on end; just five days or
so will throw up patterns, although avoid doing this if you
have any anxiety around food. Keeping a journal can also
help you see which aspects of your new regime are going
well and where there might be room for improvement. What
are your obstacles? How did you overcome them? How did

you feel? If nothing went to plan, ask yourself why … were you bored, lonely, stressed, unprepared? How can you make tomorrow better?

Your weight is not your worth

Etch this on to your brain. Put it on a post-it note. Repeat it to yourself daily.

Carbs and fast fat loss

For every gram of carbohydrate your body stores as glycogen (in the liver and muscles), it also stores 3g of water. If you go on a low-carb diet and use up your stored carbs, you lose the carb weight and the water weight. This is why low-carb diets often show significant weight loss early on, according to the scales. Be aware, though, it's largely fluid loss rather than fat loss and will usually rebound when you start eating carbs again. It's also one of the reasons a high-refined carb diet, which happens to include lots of salt – think pizza, crisps and chips – can cause water retention and that puffiness we all tend to moan about.

The bottom line

» Weight gain is multifactorial. Your genes, lifestyle, economic status, and of course hormones, all play a part.
» Slowly does it; fat loss is a marathon not a sprint.
» Plan ahead. The better prepped you are, the more likely you are to succeed: diarise fitness, make meal plans, batch cook and prepare for food emergencies.

» It's not a linear process – there will be bumps along the way. Navigate them best by reflecting on what went wrong, dusting yourself off and getting back on board.

» Don't be defined by the numbers on your scales. Your weight isn't indicative of your worth.

A Final Word

We are the first generation that will be post-menopausal for half of our lives. Let's make it count.

So now what? Good question. We've given you a lot to think about in the previous pages, so you may well want to go back and immerse yourself in the sections that resonate most. Bear in mind, as we said right at the beginning, perimenopause isn't static. It will very likely morph and shift in the months or years to come as part of your individual journey. This book is your road map and we hope it will serve as an invaluable guide to help you move forwards.

If it makes you feel any better, you've already come far. When you first picked up this book you were in a very different place to where you find yourself today. Now you have the tools, information and resources you need to navigate your way through to menopause.

So, what can you expect when you're post-menopausal and when exactly will it happen? Does it even happen if you're on HRT? Will you know when you cross over from perimenopause to post-menopause? Although these are all good questions, and although they're asked frequently, it's impossible to say with 100 per cent accuracy. On average

90 per cent of women are post-menopausal by the time they're 55. That means no periods. Less hormone disruption. More freedom.

If you're on HRT, you won't experience this, but it may be time to change from a cyclical regime to a period-free continuous one around this time. HRT doesn't stop menopause; it works to help smooth out the bumps in the journey. Don't take your eye off the prize though. You still need to continue putting in place the diet, health and lifestyle foundations we've covered, but life should be a lot more straightforward when you cross the post-menopause threshold.

The main take-home post-menopause tips, from a health and nutrition point of view are:

» We think it's time to start looking at menopause in a different light, thinking of it as a hormone-deficiency state and taking into consideration all the health risks that come with that, namely osteoporosis, dementia, diabetes and heart disease.

» HRT, when prescribed to alleviate the symptoms of menopause, is relatively safe long-term according to the Women's Health Initiative long-term randomised clinical trials in 2020.

» Menopausal weight gain is real. A third of women aged 45–50 are overweight (BMI >25) and a further third of women are obese (BMI >27). This isn't about aesthetics – being overweight increases your risk of Type 2 diabetes, hypertension, cardiovascular disease and breast cancer.

» Healthy women starting HRT in the 'window of opportunity' – i.e. within ten years of their menopause – have a reduced risk of heart disease and a reduced risk of dying from heart disease.

» Taking charge of your health and your hormones midlife can have hugely positive effects on your future health and wellbeing.

» Invest in a health audit: get your total cholesterol – triglycerides LDL ('bad' cholesterol) and HDL ('good' cholesterol) – checked by having a blood test. You might also want to test your thyroid, vitamin D and iron levels.

» Don't forget your bones. Women are at a higher risk of osteoporosis due to oestrogen loss at this time.

» Twice as many women than men develop dementia, and while more evidence is needed, it does seem that those with a family history may find the process accelerated during the perimenopause years.

Perimenopause often throws lives into stark relief. And for that we need to be thankful. It forces you to look at yourself, your environment and your future squarely in the eye. You may have blindly stumbled into perimenopause without any real understanding of what was happening, but now you're the one in the driver's seat.

And so this brings us to the end. Or is it? Hell no, not even close! In so many ways you're standing on the brink of an exhilarating new life phase. The Second Act, if you like. A time when, alongside the right attitude, knowledge and support, you can embark on the next chapter full of energy, curiosity and optimism. You know who you are, what you like, and – thankfully – how to navigate your hormones.

So, what does post-menopause look like? We hope it looks brave and unapologetic. But the truth is, it can look any way you like because this is your time to regain control, take charge of your health, refocus on what matters in life and even potentially redefine your identity. The common refrain is perimenopause marks the end of your youth and your fertility, but you can be fertile in a whole host of different ways: by starting new ventures, discovering new opportunities or simply doing things purely for yourself at last.

Despite what the media would have us all believe, midlife women are a force to be reckoned with. We're wiser, more resilient and, if this book has done its job right, more empowered to tackle the future fearlessly. We believe the stigma around menopause as a subject is slowly being chipped away, but there is still an unforgivable lack of funding, research and education. We will continue to do our bit to get the word out there via interviews, podcasts, webinars and press articles, but don't forget to play your part too. Share what you've learned, buy the women that matter in your life this book, open up about your experiences. We are the first generation that will be post-menopausal for half of our lives and what an absolute privilege it is to be here. Let's make sure it counts – for us and for all the women who come after us.

Symptoms Questionnaire

Use this list to log your symptoms, and remember, if you don't feel right, think 'perimenopause'.

Symptoms of Perimenopause	YES	NO
Period symptoms		
Shorter cycle length		
Periods irregular/missed period		
Heavy periods		
Lighter period		
Vasomotor symptoms		
Hot flushes or feeling hot		
Night sweats		
Sleep issues		
Difficulty in falling asleep		
Sleep is disrupted and broken during the night		
Waking early, typically between 3 and 5 am		
General physical symptoms		
Tired		
Palpitations		
Bloating/digestive issues		
Changes to body odour		

the perimenopause solution

Symptoms of Perimenopause	YES	NO
Weight gain		
Breast soreness/tenderness		
Joint pains		
Itchy skin		
Hair thinning or dry		
Looking old		
Dry, brittle nails		
Dental problems		
Sore mouth		
Genito-urinary symptoms		
Vaginal dryness/itching/burning		
More frequent episodes of cystitis or thrush		
Urine leaks e.g. when coughing		
Not able to hold on and needing to urinate more frequently		
Getting up in the night to pee		
Low libido/Loss of interest in sex		
Brain function		
More frequent headaches		
Brain fog		
Forgetful		
Difficulty concentrating and focusing		

Symptoms of Perimenopause	YES	NO
Psychological symptoms		
Loss of confidence		
Loss of motivation		
Feeling overwhelmed		
Loss of self esteem		
Feeling invisible/not sexy		
Mood changes		
Feeling flat		
Feeling depressed		
Mood swings/Moody		
Anxious or anxiousness		
More hypersensitive		
More irritable/rage		

References

Chapter 1

Macken, J (2017) 'How Many Eggs Do I Have?'
NICE (2017) 'Diagnosing Perimenopause and Menopause'
Avis, E and Crawford, S (2007) 'Cultural Differences in Symptoms and Attitudes Towards Menopause'
Hassan, I; Ismail, K; O'Brien, S (2004) 'PMS in the Perimenopause', National Library of Medicine, National Center for Biotechnology Information

Chapter 2

Healthline (2020) 'Why Some Women Gain Weight Around Menopause'
Kiefly, A (2018) 'Why is Dementia Different for Women?'
Sözen, T; Özisik, L; Basaran, N (2017) 'An Overview and Management of Osteoporosis'
Heart Matters (2021) 'Twice as Deadly as Breast Cancer'
Office for National Statistics 'Suicides in the UK: 2018 registrations'
NHS (2021) 'Physical Activity Guidelines for Adults Aged 19–64'
House of Commons Library (2021) 'Obesity Statistics'

Chapter 3

University of Utah (2021) 'The Natural Journey of Perimenopause'
Graham, S (2019) 'The Truth About Early Menopause'

Avis, E and Crawford, S (2007) 'Cultural Differences in Symptoms and Attitudes Towards Menopause'
Ahuja, M (2016) 'Age of Menopause and Determinants of Menopause Age: A PAN India survey by IMS', National Library of Medicine

Chapter 4

NICE (2019) 'Menopause: Diagnosis and Management'
NHS conditions (2019) 'Breast Cancer in Women'
Cancer Research UK (2021) 'Inherited Cancer Genes and Increased Cancer Risk'
British Medical Journal (2019) 'Use of Hormone Replacement Therapy and Risk of Venous Thromboembolism: nested case-control studies using the QResearch and CPRD databases'
Women's Health Concern (2017) *Understanding the Risks of Breast Cancer*

Chapter 5

Czernecka, J (2019) 'The Positive and Negative Impact of Appearance on Various Spheres of Life – the Opinions of Women and Men of Different Ages'
Obagi, S (2005) 'Why Does Skin Wrinkle With Ageing?'
Refinery29.com (2012) 'Cat Deeley is Nicest Celeb Ever'
Moran, C (2020) 'Caitlin Moran: this is what a feminist who has botox looks like'

Chapter 6

Cohen, L; Soares, C; Joffe, H (2019) 'Diagnosis and Management of Mood Disorders During the Menopausal Transition'
Office for National Statistics 'Divorces in England and Wales: 2017'

Bromberger, J; Epperson, C (2018) 'Depression During and After the Perimenopause: impact of hormones, genetics, and environmental determinants of disease'

MIND (2021) 'Mental Health Problems – an Introduction'

NICE (2019) 'Menopause: diagnosis and management'

MIND (2021) 'St John's Wort – Hypericum perforatum'

Kulkarni, J (2018) 'Perimenopausal Depression – an Under-Recognised Entity'

Women's Health Concerns (2017) 'New Survey Highlights Impact of the Menopause on Every Aspect of Women's Lives in the UK'

Garcia, M; Umberson, D (2019) 'Marital Strain and Psychological Distress in Same-Sex and Different-Sex Couples'

Chapter 7

England, C (2016) 'Women Suffering from Loss of Sexual Desire Should be Offered Testosterone on the NHS', *Independent*

Goldstein, I et al. (2016) 'Hypoactive Sexual Desire Disorder'

Warnock, J (2002) 'Female Hypoactive Sexual Desire Disorder: epidemiology, diagnosis and treatment'

Goldstein, I et al. (2017) 'Hypoactive Sexual Desire Disorder: International Society for the Study of Women's Sexual Health (ISSWSH) Expert Consensus Panel review'

Chapter 8

Whelan, E et al. (1990) 'Menstrual and Reproductive Characteristics and Age at Natural Menopause'

Gooley, J et al. (2001) 'Exposure to Room Light Before Bedtime Suppresses Melatonin Onset and Shortens Melatonin Duration in Humans'

Kimberly, B and Phelps, J (2009) 'Amber Lenses to Block Blue Light and Improve Sleep: a randomised trial'

Mullen, B et al. (2008) 'Exploring the Safety and Therapeutic Effects of Deep Pressure Stimulation Using a Weighted Blanket'

The Vegan Society, www.vegansociety.com

Harvey, A and Farrell, C (2003) 'The Efficacy of a Pennebaker-like Writing Intervention for Poor Sleepers'

Scullin, M et al. (2018) 'The Effects of Bedtime Writing on Difficulty Falling Asleep'

Sarris, J et al. (2018) 'L-theanine in the Adjunctive Treatment of Generalized Anxiety Disorder: a double-blind, randomised, placebo-controlled trial'

Inagawa, K et al. (2006) 'Subjective Effects of Glycine Ingestion Before Bedtime on Sleep'

Kawai, N et al. (2015) 'The Sleep Promoting and Hypothermic Effects of Glycine'

Chapter 9

ITV News (2016) 'Quarter of Women Going Through Menopause "Considered Leaving Work"'

The School of Life (2021) 'How Your Job Shapes Your Identity'

Robins, E (2021) 'The Secret Benefit of Routines. It Won't Surprise You'.

Clark, D (2021) 'Number of Female Held CEO Positions in FTSE Companies in the United Kingdom (UK) as of June 2019'

GOV.UK (2021) 'Flexible Working'

Garlick, D (2020) 'Employment Law and Menopause'

Gaskell, A (2020) 'Productivity in Times of Covid'

Madgavker, A et al. (2020) 'COVID-19 and Gender Equality: countering the regressive effects'

Chapter 10

Kris-Etherton, P et al. (2001) 'Lyon Diet Heart Study' diabetes.co.uk, accessed 2020

De Alzaa, F et al. (2018) 'Evaluation of Chemical and Physical Changes in Different Commercial Oils during Heating'

Samieri, C et al. (2013) 'The Association between Dietary Patterns at Midlife and Health and Ageing'

Aune, D et al. (2017) 'Fruit and Vegetable Intake and the Risk of Cardiovascular Disease, Total Cancer and All-Cause Mortality – a Systematic Review'

Rickman, JC et al. (2007) 'Nutritional Comparison of Fresh, Frozen and Canned Fruits and Vegetables'

Paddon-Jones, D (2010) 'Dietary Protein Recommendations and the Prevention of Sarcopenia'

Berg, JM and Tymoczko, JL, *Biochemistry*, New York, 2002, 5th edition

nutrition.org.uk, accessed December 2020

Xu, Y et al. (2018) 'Wholegrain Diet Reduces Systemic Inflammation'

Lillioja, S et al. (2014) 'Wholegrains, Type 2 Diabetes, Coronary Heart Disease and Hypertension'

Chapter 11

Dreno, B (2001) 'Multicenter Randomized Comparative Double-blind Controlled Clinical Trial of the Safety and Efficacy of Zinc Gluconate versus Minocycline Hydrochloride in the Treatment of Inflammatory Acne Vulgaris'

Porru, D (2014) 'Oral D-mannose in Recurrent Urinary Tract Infections in Women: a pilot study'

Chang, C, et al. (2010) 'Kiwifruit Improves Bowel Function in Patients with Irritable Bowel Syndrome with Constipation'

Gagnier, J (2001) 'The Therapeutic Potential of Melatonin in Migraines and other Headache Types'

Rozen, TD (2002) 'Open Label Trial of Coenzyme Q10 as a Migraine Preventive'

Boehnke, C et al. (2004) 'High Dose Riboflavin is Efficacious in Migraine Prophylaxis'

Hartman, TJ (2016) 'Alcohol Consumption and Urinary Oestrogens and Oestrogen Metabolites'

Franco, O et al. (2016) 'Use of Plant-Based Therapies and Menopausal Symptoms – A Systematic Review and Meta-analysis'

Daily, J. et al. (2016) 'Efficacy of Turmeric Extracts and Curcumin for Alleviating Joint Arthritis: a systematic review and meta-analysis of randomised clinical trials'

Suchonwanit, P. (2019) 'Minoxidil and Its Use in Hair Disorders: a review'

Larmo, P (2014) 'Effects of Sea Buckthorn Oil Intake on Vaginal Atrophy in Postmenopausal Women: a randomized, double-blind, placebo-controlled study'

Chapter 12

Askarova, S et al. (2020) 'The Links Between the Gut Microbiome, Ageing, Modern Lifestyle and Alzheimer's Disease'

Kwa, M et al. (2016) 'The Intestinal Microbiome and Estrogen Positive Female Breast Cancer'

Baothman, O et al. (2016) 'The Role of Gut Microbiota in the Development of Obesity and Diabetes'

Blottiere, H et al (2015) 'The Influence of Diet on the Gut Microbiota and Its Consequences for Health'

Dao, M et al. (2015) 'Akkermansia Muciniphilia and Improved Metabolic Health During a Dietary Intervention in Obesity' americangut.org, accessed 2020

Kwa, M. et al. (2016) 'The Intestinal Microbiome and Estrogen Receptor – Positive Female Breast Cancer'

Chapter 13

Schuch, F (2016) 'Exercise as a Treatment for Depression: a meta-analysis adjusting for publication bias'

Guthrie, J (2005) 'Hot Flushes During the Menopause Transition: a longitudinal study in Australian-born women'

Bailey, T et al. (2015) 'Exercise Training Reduces the Acute Physiological Severity of Post-menopausal Hot Flushes'

Woods, R et al. (2019) 'Association of Lean Body Mass to Menopausal Symptoms: the study of women's health across the nation'

Eriksen, W and Bruusgaard, D (2004) 'Do Physical Leisure Time Activities Prevent Fatigue? A 15-month prospective study of nurses' aides.'

King, A et al. (1997) 'Moderate-intensity Exercise and Self-rated Quality of Sleep in Older Adults: a randomized controlled trial'

Benedetti, M et al. (2018) 'The Effectiveness of Physical Exercise on Bone Density in Osteoporotic Patients'

Chlebowski, R (2013) 'Nutrition and Physical Activity Influence on Breast Cancer Incidence and Outcome'

Schuch, F et al. (2016) 'Exercise as a Treatment for Depression: a meta-analysis adjusting for publication bias'

Hu, F et al. (2000) 'Physical Activity and Risk of Stroke in Women'

Hildebrand, J et al. (2013) 'Recreational Physical Activity and Leisure-time Sitting in Relation to Postmenopausal Breast Cancer Risk'

Matthews, C et al. (2018) 'Amount and Intensity of Leisure Time Physical Activity and Lower Cancer Risk'

Hanson, S and Jones, A (2015) 'Is there Evidence that Walking Groups have Health Benefits? A Systematic Review and Meta-analysis.'

Oppezzo, M and Schwartz, D (2014) 'Give Your Ideas Some Legs. The Positive Effects of Walking on Creativity.'

Miller, J and Krizan, Z (2016) 'Walking Facilitates Positive Affect (Even When Expecting the Opposite)'

Nieman, D et al. (2011) 'Upper Respiratory Tract Infection is Reduced in Physically Fit and Active Adults'

Wang, W et al. (2020) 'The Effect of Yoga on Sleep Quality and Insomnia in Women with Sleep Problems: a systematic review and meta-analysis'

Levine, J et al. (1999) 'Role of Non-exercise Activity Thermogenesis in Resistance to Fat Gain in Humans'

https://www.nhs.uk/live-well/exercise/why-sitting-too-much-is-bad-for-us/, accessed 2020

Vallance, J et al. (2018) 'Evaluating the Evidence on Sitting, Smoking, and Health: is sitting really the new smoking?'

Chapter 14

Hróbjartsson, A and Gøtzsche, PC (2010) 'Placebo Interventions for All Clinical Conditions'

Buijze, G et al. (2016) 'The Effect of Cold Showering on Health and Work: a randomized controlled trial'

Costantino, D et al. (2009) 'Metabolic and Hormonal Effects of Myo-inositol in Women with Polycystic Ovary Syndrome: a double-blind trial'

Fortmann, SP et al. (2013) 'Vitamin and Mineral Supplements in the Primary Prevention of Cardiovascular Disease and Cancer'

Blessing, E et al. (2015) 'Cannabidiol as a Potential Treatment for Anxiety Disorders'

Skelley, J et al. (2019) 'Use of Cannabidiol in Anxiety and Anxiety-related Disorders'

Kuhathasan, N et al. (2019) 'The Use of Cannabinoids for Sleep: a critical review on clinical trials'

Chapter 15

Health Survey for England, http://healthsurvey.hscic.gov.uk/data-visualisation/data-visualisation/explore-the-trends/weight.aspx

Blankert, T and Hamstra, R (2016) 'Imagining Success: multiple achievement goals and the effectiveness of imagery'

Dalle Grave, R et al. (2005) 'Weight Loss Expectations in Obese Patients and Treatment Attrition: an observational multicenter study'

Final word

The Collaborative Group on Hormonal Factors in Breast Cancer (2019)

Further Resources

Websites

emmabardwell.com

theharperclinic.com

bacp.co.uk – British Association for Counselling and Psychotherapy

beateatingdisorders.org.uk – Beat Eating Disorders

coppafeel.org – Breast Cancer

daisynetwork.org – The Daisy Network (premature and early menopause support)

endometriosis-uk.org – Endometriosis UK

eveappeal.org.uk – Gynaecological Cancer

histamineintolerance.org.uk – Histamine Intolerance

nimh.org.uk – National Institute of Medical Herbalists

pms.org.uk – National Association for Premenstrual Syndromes (NAPS)

sleepfoundation.org – Sleep Foundation

stonewall.org.uk – Stonewall (LGBT advice and support)

thebms.org.uk – The British Menopause Society

Recommended books

Oestrogen Matters: Why Taking Hormones in Menopause Can Improve Women's Well-Being and Lengthen Their Lives – Without Raising the Risk of Breast Cancer by Avrum Bluming

The Worry Trick: How Your Brain Tricks You into Expecting the Worst and What You Can Do About It by David A. Carbonell

Invisible Women: Exposing Data Bias in a World Designed for Men by Caroline Criado Perez

The Unexpected Joy of Being Sober: Discovering a Happy, Healthy, Wealthy Alcohol-free Life by Catherine Gray

The Circadian Code: Lose Weight, Supercharge Your Energy and Sleep Well Every Night by Dr Satchin Panda

How To Break Up With Your Phone: The 30-Day Plan to Take Back Your Life by Catherine Price

Acknowledgements

Our heartfelt thanks go to all the team at Penguin Random House for recognising the need for this book and giving us the opportunity to bring our vision to life. A special mention to our agent, Valeria Huerta, who instantly got the whole concept and our passion to put it into print. And thanks to our clients and patients, who so graciously shared their stories and experiences anonymously.

Shahzadi: Thanks to all those along the way who have believed in me, especially my daughter who told me 'it was my time to shine'.

Emma: Thanks to Raf for keeping the kids alive while I locked myself in my room to write. I couldn't have done this without your support. And to my rebel girls, Aggie and Margot, for tolerating the endless chat about dry vaginas: there is officially nothing you don't know about perimenopause. I'm singling out Sue, Jim and Nives for making life infinitely better and my tribe of brilliant cheerleaders – you know who you are – for always believing in me. Dr Natalia Spierings is a skin genius, Beth Jackson-Edwards has wise eyes and no one knows herbs like Marion Colledge – your respective inputs were invaluable.

Finally, Simon ... you said I could do it and I did. Not a day goes by when I don't think about you.

Index

Page references in *italics* indicate images.